Contents

Acknowledgements

Many thanks go to:

Avril Nicholl, Editor of *Speech & Language Therapy in Practice*, who was happy to lend her support to the original body of articles printed in her magazine, and then kindly allowed them to be included in this book.

Julia Meyer, SLT assistant and friend, who helped to create some of these unusual and funny games.

The students at: William Morris House Camphill Community, Stroud College and Ruskin Mill College, who inspired all of these games, and the staff there, who have created environments in which communication work can flourish.

Hilary Whates of Speechmark, for her continued encouragement.

My husband Peter Roberts for his technical and IT support.

Tom Roberts for his help with the Ambiguity chapter.

Amy Gjoci for extra material included in several games.

Faith Roberts for proofreading and support.

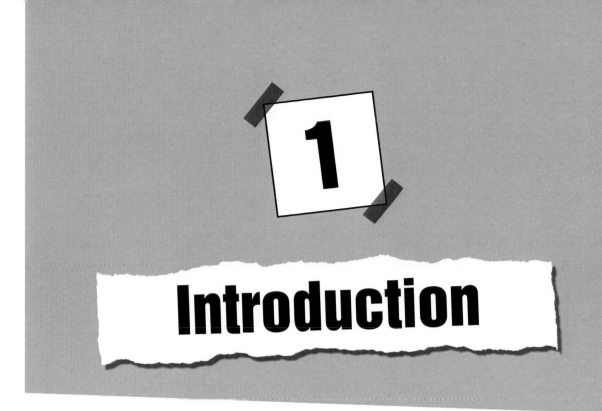

Introduction

For a long time I have been waiting for someone to write a book containing all sorts of cheap but useful ideas for enlivening and extending Speech and Language Therapy (SLT) sessions.

In my clinic I have always had many boxes of lovely photo cards and games. However, there is sometimes not quite the right resource for a particular client or group, or if there is, it is beyond the SLT purse. With all the talented therapy writers and resource makers creating great books and games I was sure that someone would write something for the therapist on a budget. Nobody did, so I have found myself attempting to fill this gap, and here is a collection of ideas that should provide you with new resources for very little money.

Good practice involves careful diagnosis and planning. To augment the well-established and structured programmes of therapy that speech and language therapists use, I have discovered four principles that can make for better therapeutic outcomes:

1 Most clients will respond more effectively if they feel they 'own' their therapy by being involved in making the materials they will use, so that the creative process becomes part of the therapy.

2 Sitting alongside clients making an item lends an atmosphere of working at their therapy together, giving guidance. This seating arrangement also reduces the chances of too much eye contact, which is helpful for some people who have a diagnosis on the autism spectrum.

3 Therapy is vastly improved when it is good fun, and preferably humorous. Clients will usually want to attend their next session if they have left the previous one with the warm glow of having had a good laugh. (And don't neglect yourself – if you have had fun in a session you will be a happier therapist!)

4 Sometimes clients make for themselves (or with a little help) something they like and want to keep. Such an item will be a pleasant reminder of something learned during their therapy, and might encourage them to return to therapy after a break.

I have always wished that cartoon drawing had been a module of my SLT training, and that *Blue Peter* studies had been another, but actually you don't need to be a great artist or craftsperson to create these games and activities. Also, you don't need huge quantities of spare time to make most of the items, especially if you can get organised with the equipment you need all in one go. I have provided a basic shopping list to help you get started.

Some of the games and activities address particular communication themes, for example, listening techniques or friendship skills, while others cover several areas simultaneously. I have divided the book into chapters according to either the skill area being addressed or the way in which the items can be used.

It is worth noting that although many of the activities and games note an appropriate age level, most of them can in fact be adapted for different groups just by presenting them in different ways – for example, a board game, however simple, can appeal to adults if the decoration is mature, or tailored to a particular interest. You have control over this process, so there is another advantage to producing your own equipment rather than buying ready-made items.

This book is essentially a body of practical ideas for you to use in your therapy, based on my experiences. Most chapters are concerned with an aspect of therapy, and begin with an introduction. Some references are included, and these indicate some of my own background reading, as well as forming a body of recommended reading, should you wish to further your knowledge in any particular area.

Above all, this book seeks to inspire you with confidence to invent your own games and activities, tailored to your clients and clinical settings.

Standard items to have in your cupboard

- A4 and A5 paper and coloured card.
- Pens, felt tip pens, pencils and sharpener.
- Right- and left-handed scissors.
- Glues (Pritt Stick and PVA), Sellotape and Blu-Tack.
- Ruler.
- Blank business cards, index cards and blank postcards.
- 'Taskmaster' blank playing cards.
- Flipchart paper rolls (needed for larger sheets, so ends of rolls are fine).

Also useful

- Box of odd, unwanted (even broken but safe) plastic, metal or wooden items or parts of items.
- Box of scraps of different fabrics.

 Speechmark

- Watercolour paints in tubes.

- Upholsterer's foam of 75mm thickness, preferably cut into 75mm cubes.

- Planned timber, 50mm by 50mm, preferably cut into 50mm lengths to form cubes.

- Empty plastic drinks bottles.

- Lining paper, sold in DIY shops alongside wallpaper. It is flat and white or cream, and quite strong.

- Wire coat hangers and picture hooks for displaying your clients' work and decorating the room.

- Defunct boxes of Scrabble, often to be found at car boot sales and on markets – it's the tiles you are after, and it doesn't necessarily matter if it is not a full set.

- The cheapest possible baking parchment you can find. Don't confuse baking parchment with greaseproof paper; baking parchment will not stick, whereas greaseproof will.

Save

- Shoe boxes – for storage.

- Packaging trays from packs of small plants, or similar from some types of biscuits and chocolates.

- Jokes from crackers (however groan-making you think they are!).

- Dented or otherwise damaged toy cars.

Facilities needed or desirable

- Wall space.

- A shelf where you can leave items that your clients have made while the glue or paint dries.

- Fibreboard notice boards.

- Blackboard.

- Access to a PC and photocopier.

- Access to a paper guillotine.

Speechmark

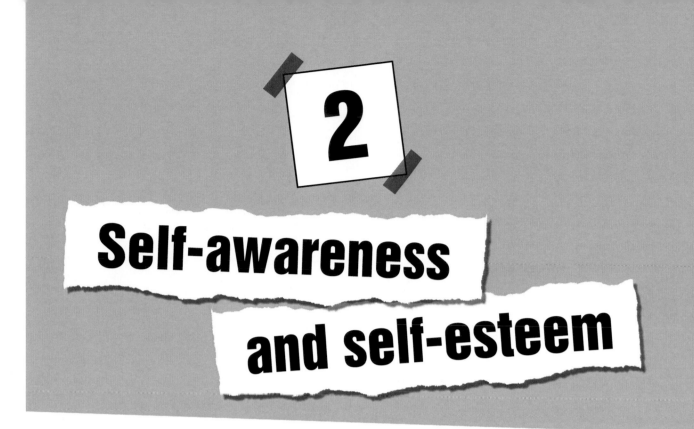

2

Self-awareness and self-esteem

Raising someone's self-esteem can be a long and uphill task, but here you will have beads, paint, tee-shirts and paper chains to help you!

Therapists often see clients who have experienced years of not being understood, or of misunderstanding others. Such clients may arrive at our clinics not only with their given, named and particular diagnoses but also having grafted on their own coping strategies, with varying degrees of success.

Sometimes a client's strategies may include avoiding situations where they might have to communicate with others, retreating into timidity or silence and isolation. Perhaps they are now disillusioned with the whole idea of talking with others, and regard themselves as poor communicators, and/or not worth talking to. They may have decided that, for example, it would be better not to put up their hand to answer a question in class, or older clients may prefer not to try to offer an opinion in a conversation, or to take the first tentative steps in forming a relationship.

On the other hand, they may try putting on a brave face, ignoring other people's comments, and attempting to convey that their ways are equal or superior to everyone else's. This may well be misinterpreted by others as arrogance, with again the result of them becoming isolated.

Occasionally we encounter the type of client who has adopted a role of being the class or community clown, and while sometimes this role can be carried off successfully, there is often the risk of being laughed *at* rather than *with*, which can lead to a situation where they are bullied.

In some cases these feelings of worthlessness, the social isolation, the desire not to communicate with others or being bullied may become so severe that help from other professionals – counsellors, psychotherapists, and so on – may be needed. We need to be sensitive and make appropriate referrals when necessary.

However, here are some ideas to help when the case is not so severe, or for after or alongside other therapies.

'All about me' boxes

This is a self-awareness activity. It is best done over several sessions, taking time to complete the boxes to a good finish and talk them through. You can carry out this activity with just one client, or in a group.

A word of warning: this activity should be carried out in a light-hearted atmosphere, you are not trying to be a psychotherapist.

My advice is to make a box about yourself before the session, which you are prepared to open to reveal the contents. However, you should state clearly to your clients that they will not have to reveal the contents of their boxes to others if they do not wish to.

Materials needed

- Small (about 75mm x 75mm x 25mm) plain-coloured cardboard boxes, available from craft shops. The best sorts have a frame within the lid. If you really cannot run to that expense, then the small individual cereal boxes sold in packs are a good substitute, but you or your clients will need to paint them white before decorating, and make a neat opening at one end (and of course you have to remove the contents first!).
- A photo of your client.
- Felt tip pens.
- Small pieces of paper or card.
- Sticky tape.
- Varnish.
- Magazines.

Making your boxes

Use felt tip pens to decorate the outside of the box. Decorations can include images and words to show the world what this person is good at, or likes to do, and should include their first name. If your client is happy to do so, they will stick their photo on the lid of the box, within the frame. This part is on view, for others to inspect.

Some clients prefer to stick on pictures from magazines rather than their own drawings, so you or they will need to supply magazines which interest them – football, fishing, sewing, fashion magazines and so forth are all easily available. If they would like to use that approach, then – in an art of decorating known as decoupage – pictures can be cut or torn out, then stuck on the box, perhaps building up and overlapping the images. Then the box will need to be varnished (acrylic gel varnish is good), using several coats, so that the 'stuck on', multiple sources, appearance is lost.

Inside the box your client will place small pieces of paper or card with words on to describe their secrets, fears, disappointments, dreams, and so on. Some clients may like to have some help in writing down their thoughts, and some may like to chat about the contents with you. It is important for the clients to be sure that the boxes are kept in a secure place, and that you will not look inside without their permission. When they have completely finished making the boxes they may like to seal them with tape, or perhaps with attractive stickers.

Variation

This is good for a group setting. Together, each client begins writing on the pieces of paper or card that will go inside their box, starting with some less 'sensitive' topics, for example, preferences (favoured holiday resorts, music, types of food, best ever film, etc), or aspects of the clients' biographies (birthday, place where their childhood was spent, schooling, etc). If they are all willing, try this: pool all of the cards, and take turns to pick one out and guess who wrote it, before placing it in its owner's box. This can form a pleasant 'getting-to-know-you' session in the clinic. Later, cards with more private thoughts can be placed in the box without others seeing.

Please note: try to create an atmosphere where clients are happy to chat about the contents of their boxes, but be aware that occasionally disclosures are made that might need to be referred to another professional. My advice is to warn clients that anything said in the session by one member of the group must not be repeated by another member outside of the session. You yourself, however, should not promise to keep secrets, because you might hear a disclosure that needs action urgently from another professional.

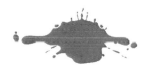

'How I help people' poster

This is useful for self-esteem building, also self-awareness or awareness of others, and as a background to friendship skills, and it can make a good wall decoration.

Materials needed

- Paper.
- Photocopier.
- Pens.
- White stickers.

Making the poster

Place your own, or your client's, hand on the platen of the photocopier. Now close the lid and preferably cover it with a cloth to exclude as much daylight as possible. Take a photocopy and then copy this several times once you are satisfied with the image, as these copies are useful for several different posters. Store the spares flat. Older teenagers seem to like to photocopy their own hands. Don't worry if they are wearing jewellery or watches, as these photocopy surprisingly well, and add individuality.

If you have any health and safety qualms about photocopying clients' hands then you, or they, can draw around their hands instead.

Procedure

Use the hand image to make an insightful and esteem-raising poster. Head the poster 'How I help' or 'As a friend I ...'

Fill in a 'quality' or two in each finger and thumb, or in the palm. You may need to add small white stickers if the palm is too dark on the photocopy.

The 'qualities' written on the poster can be quite simple, for example, for the 'How I help' version, the statement might be: 'I give out the biscuits', 'I carry people's books', or 'I open the window for my houseparent'.

For the 'Friend' poster, they might write: 'I smile at my friend', 'I share chocolate', 'I remember birthdays', or 'I let my friend choose which film we are going to see'.

For a group setting you could cut out the hands and stick them on to a larger sheet as if reaching for each other.

Variation

Consider using the other copies for similar posters, for example, 'My strengths', 'My hobbies' or 'My favourite sports'. We made a mobile of 'My preferences' hand photocopies by sticking them on to stiff card – so that we could use both sides. We then tied them to crossed sticks, and suspended the whole thing from the ceiling.

Posters and mobiles like these can be a good way to decorate your clinic. For other decoration ideas please see Chapter 15 'Wallcharts and decorations'.

Paint splotch predictions

This is a self-awareness activity, for just one client or for a group. Please be aware that paint in tubes does squirt! You may need to cover the table with newspaper, and provide aprons, old tee-shirts or large paper napkins to protect clients' clothes.

Materials needed

- Heavyweight A4 paper. 100gm photocopy paper is adequate, but 135gm cartridge paper would be even better.

- Watercolour paints in tubes, preferably avoiding browns and black unless you are working with Goth clients.

- Pens.

- Scissors.

Making the splotches

Each client should make a wish to do with their current communication target, for example, 'I want to get better at using the phone', 'I want to make a friend' or 'I want to improve at smiling at people'. Try to encourage realistic targets that could be achieved within the course of therapy. These targets are written a little way above the bottom of the paper, which can be landscape or portrait way round.

The paper is now folded down the middle and the paper opened up again.

Small blobs of different colours of paint are squeezed fairly closely together in the upper part of the centre fold, that is, away from the written prediction. Now the paper is refolded and pressed flat, 'squidging' the paint outwards from the fold, and mixing the colours together a little.

Unfold your paper and here is an instant work of art with a pleasing symmetry, which you can 'interpret' together. Perhaps you can see a telephone or a bit of cable there, or a pair of shaking hands, or a smile. You may have to be very imaginative, but you should be able to see something, that can be a prediction that the target can be achieved.

If possible, make a frame for each picture by cutting a large rectangular hole into another sheet of paper, but take care that the written wish is still visible. These make colourful wall displays en masse and can be taken down and evaluated together at the end of the course – were the predictors right? Maybe things are going the way the predictor said, but you interpreted the time for improvement wrongly. You should of course engineer things so that something positive can be celebrated.

Variation

After making the splotches, use them as a discussion tool to help you and the client to decide which area should be worked on next.

We have used them for a fun activity in January, to predict something general that might happen during the year.

You might also want to use these pictures as motivational tools: 'Look, your paint splotch prediction says that you will have made a good /g/ sound by half-term; you are already quite good at it so maybe if we just do a little more work on it you'll be able to say you are good at predicting.'

For other motivation ideas please see Chapter 11 'Motivating your clients'.

Paint splotch pictures also make good decorations. For other decoration ideas please see Chapter 15 'Wallcharts and decorations'.

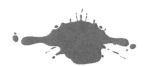

'Same and different' chains

People with communication disorders, especially those on the autism spectrum, often express feelings of low self-esteem, mentioning that they are not like other people. This activity is a pressure-free way for your clients to consider and celebrate (a) people's similarities, and (b) their unique qualities. If you have a wall available, it also makes a rather good display, with especially high impact if there are several together.

Materials needed

- Long strips of paper about 10–15cm wide; lining wallpaper cut lengthways into three will be tough, cheap and long.

- Good scissors (left-handed scissors are great for those who need them, and a worthwhile investment).

- Felt tip pens, thin coloured tissue paper, or sticky paper or shapes, for decorating the chains.

Making your chain

Fold your strip of paper into a concertina. You will probably be able to cut through about six layers of paper at a time (some clients may not be able to do so many), and each flat area will need to be big enough to draw a person on.

Draw the outline of a person (two-dimensional, not a 'stick person') on the front. A key point to make if your clients are making these themselves is that the hands (or elbows if hands are on hips), and/or outer edges of skirt, hat or shoes must stretch to the outside edge to create joining points. Now cut out through all the layers, making sure you don't cut through the joining points – otherwise you will end up with a lot of separate paper people rather than a chain. If you create more than one joining point the chain will be stronger. Have some female chains and some male ones.

Once the paper shapes have been cut out and opened up you will be able to discuss how people in general are similar to look at, and you can talk about our other similarities and emphasise our common humanity. You might also want to mention straight away that if we were all exactly the same, life would be boring. Stick one of these chains that show human similarities on the wall.

Now you can move on to the interesting fact of uniqueness or individuality, by decorating the people in another paper chain, being sure to make some female and some male, of various ethnicities, hair colour, some with glasses or hearing aids and so on, and of varying ages. As well as talking about external appearance, you might want to mention people's differing preferences, lifestyles, and so forth, and could add words to the cut-outs' bodies to indicate these differences.

It is important to make it clear that we are all different, and that it's fine to be as we are.

Variation

If you widen the concertinas so that you can fit in two people on the front, holding hands, you can make one more obviously female and one more male, or one fatter and one taller, or one older and one younger, and so on, creating lots of 'opposites pairs'. You can also add speech bubbles, either as a part of the cut-out, or separately by attaching those useful speech bubble-shaped Post-it notes.

Self-awareness beads

This is a good way for a group of children or teenagers to improve their self-awareness in a private or semi-private way. Girls particularly like this activity, but some boys seem to be quite happy to make these too, especially if the beads are brownish, or edged in a dark colour.

Materials needed

- Thin knitting needles or strong wire, or meat skewers with the ends made safe by rounding off the points with a file.
- White or coloured paper.
- Small, preferably wooden, beads from a craft shop (make sure they have a biggish threading hole that will fit on to your needle, wire or skewer).
- PVA glue.
- Felt tips.
- Varnish (I recommend the acrylic type).
- Scissors.
- Narrow elastic (craft shops sell elastic especially designed for threading beads; It's best to buy the thinnest type available).
- Needles that will be narrow enough to fit through the holes, yet with wide enough eyes to accommodate the elastic.
- Baking parchment (not greaseproof paper).
- Envelopes.
- Packaging trays from chocolates or small plants.

Procedure

Cut long narrow triangles – about 10cm (4in) long and 2cm (1¾in) wide, tapering to a point. (You may need to do this yourself if your clients have trouble with their fine motor skills.)

Colour the very outermost edges of the tapered point of each triangle.

Write along the triangle anything of interest about yourself. If you want to keep the information a secret you write it at the fatter end of the triangle, but if you are prepared to share a little of your disclosure you put it towards the thinner end. You will need to use very small writing! Alternatively you could add tiny decorations – hearts, smiley faces, stars and so on are quite popular.

Turn the triangles writing and decorated side down and apply paste along the length of the other side.

Place the knitting needle or wire across the fat end of the triangle and roll it up from the fat end. You should end up with a bead that is oval and ridged like a croissant – because that is exactly how they roll up croissants, from the fat end. You should be able to make several beads on one needle.

A few trials are advisable first before you spring it on your clients – you will soon see how much of the writing is visible.

Now you must leave the beads to dry until your next session.

Ideally you would varnish the beads before use as this will prevent them from unrolling, and make them last much longer, but that means you will have to repeat the drying process. (You might be able to do this between sessions for the clients.) Just use a small amount of varnish and place on baking parchment where they won't stick. Once dry, store them in individual envelopes, or in the indented packaging trays that some small plants, biscuits and chocolates come in, so that each client's beads are separate.

Now comes the interesting bit – threading the beads on to the elastic, interspersing the made ones with the ready-made variety that you have bought. You can make either a necklace or a bracelet.

The clients should find that they have something at the end they can actually wear.

Tee-shirt activity

This is a more expensive activity, but was very much enjoyed by our clients. You might ask for contributions towards the cost. There are some very cheap tee-shirts on the high street nowadays, but wherever you buy them, the cotton variety seems to work best.

The activity is best done in a group as a sociable activity, but you will need an assistant.

The idea is to decorate the tee-shirts as a form of self-expression, showing the clients' main interests. You may need to help the clients with the task, so that they end up with something they would wear. However, you may find, as we did, that they are very artistic and don't need much help.

Materials needed

- Cheap cotton tee-shirts, or little strappy tops – one for each client; white ones make the most impact.

- Fabric paints and pens in several colours.

- Large rigid plastic stencils can be quite useful, if the clients would like to do a lot of lettering and want it to be precise.

- Baking parchment.

- Somewhere large and flat to store the shirts while they dry.

- Large pieces of scrap paper to try out designs on and to practise squeezing out the fabric paints.

- A large tray or piece of hardboard for each client.

- Pencils.

Procedure

It's really best to wash (or for the clients to wash) the tee-shirts first to get rid of any fabric finish, as then the decoration will stick on better. When you wash them, avoid fabric conditioner, and hang them up to keep them flat.

First you need to make lists of your clients' interests. We had horse riding, various pop bands and other music, dolphins, cats and dogs, cookery, and many more. They will be decorating their own shirts rather than each other's, so it doesn't matter how individual their ideas are – train timetables are acceptable if that's what turns you on! Not all the ideas will be easy to make into pictures; some can be left as lettering.

The clients should outline their designs in pencil on paper first, not straight on to the fabric. That way you can check whether the design will actually fit. Simple outlines and lettering work best, also neatly measured grids with small objects or lettering in each mini-square look good. The neck or cuffs can be accentuated with lines, dots, zigzags, and so on.

It is wise to let the clients try out the feel and effect of the fabric pens on some paper before using them on the shirts.

Before you start decorating the shirts, place them on pieces of hardboard or large trays to keep them flat. Also, insert some paper (baking parchment for preference, as it doesn't stick) between the layers of the garment to prevent the colours leaking through to the back.

Copy your design from the pencil-and-paper prototype, starting at the top to avoid smudging it. Warning – don't fold it or turn it over while it is wet; keep it flat until dry. If they want to decorate the back as well as the front of the garment you will need to do the second side in the next session.

Variations

There is a type of glue that you spread on to purchased photocopied designs, and then iron on. We found this a good idea for some, but you need to follow the instructions carefully, otherwise the paper sticks on and is hard to shift. If you use this method you need to complete the ironing part of the process before adding any other fabric pen designs, as some fabric pens are heat intolerant. Also with this version you need to work harder to clarify the point that the transfers they choose are connected with their interests, not just random images.

A 'fashion show' might add to the proceedings if clients are willing!

Other ideas for raising self-awareness and self-esteem

Please see also:

1 'Fields of interest' in Chapter 15 'Wallcharts and decorations'.

2 'Interaction paper chains for Christmas' in Chapter 15 'Wallcharts and decorations'.

3 'Face-out descriptions' in Chapter 3 'Awareness of others'.

4 'Incredible powers' in Chapter 7 'Lateral thinking'.

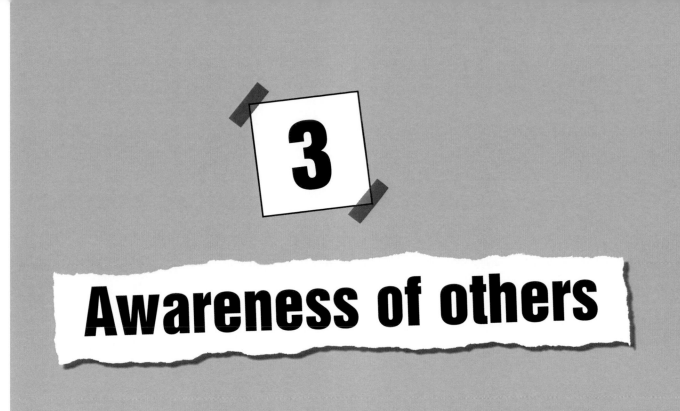

Awareness of others

Some of our clients make mistakes in the ways that they interact with others, perhaps interrupting, ignoring, arguing inappropriately, and so forth.

Sometimes these mistakes may be connected with a difficulty in recognising that other people, with their different opinions and preferences, can still be fine and acceptable friends. They may not understand ideas about 'Thank goodness we're all different' or 'Wouldn't life be boring if we were all the same' or '*Vive la* différence!'

This difficulty in tolerating other people's different ideas can lead to arguments and may get our clients labelled as 'awkward customers'. This in turn may make socialising difficult, leaving them sidelined, or without friends.

An underlying skill for understanding and tolerating others is first to notice people's qualities – their appearance, including clothes, the gestures that they use and any expressions or vocabulary they frequently use. A tip for improving people's ability to look and listen in this way is to watch part of a TV 'impressions' show, either together as a group, or as 'homework'. Sometimes it is easier to work out how for example, a politician talks or walks, after you have seen this filtered or exaggerated via a comic impressionist. Learning to look and listen should also help clients to hear and understand conversations and facial expressions.

This chapter offers some ideas for activities to help with accepting other people, even aiming to help clients begin to enjoy other people's differing opinions.

Customised Guess Who

This is a fun way for clients to learn to put names to faces, especially in a new environment.

Materials needed

- One Guess Who game, available from most toyshops, or you may have an old one available. (You could make one, but the effort will be great, and the end result may be less professional than your client is used to.)

- Photos of all those people whose names and faces you want your clients to learn. You will need three copies of each photo. You need enough different photos to fill the spaces on the flip-up board (mine has 20). Where I work we have a student handbook which contains conveniently sized photos of all the staff, but you might have to take the photos yourself, or perhaps the clients could do this as a project. It is easy to update the photos when staff move on. Warning – don't take or use pictures of students for this game.

- Card or stiff paper.

- Small labels.

Making your game

Pop out all the original pictures from both boards. Put these and the loose cards to one side and reserve for later replacement if you want to change back.

Use an original picture as a template to draw around for a good fit in the slot on the flip-up board.

Simply put your new pictures in place of the originals, labelling them with their names as you go. You must have the same selection of photos on each board, but not in the same positions. If the photos are on reasonably stiff paper you won't need to stick them on to a backing, but bear in mind that the reverse of the card looks better if it is blank, so you might want to stick the photos on to paper.

The third set of photos is needed for the loose cards, and these can be stuck on to the card or stiff paper so that the image cannot be seen from the reverse side. These pictures will also all need name labels. For a professional effect you could laminate them; they will also last much longer that way.

How to play

Each of the two players takes one of the loose cards from the selection, which should all have been turned face down. They place it in their card stand, turning it away from their opponent.

If you don't have the original rules from the box this is what you do: the idea is for the opponents to guess who is shown on the other person's card, by progressively discounting

Speechmark

'wrong' pictures. So they take it in turns to ask a general question and turn down the cards on their own board that do not fit the description.

For example; ask whether the person on the opponent's chosen photo has facial hair. If the answer is negative then all the pictures of men with moustaches and/or beards are turned down. If the answer is positive, that is, if he does have facial hair, then all of the photos showing men without facial hair are turned down. It may take a while for clients to learn that they will find the answer more quickly if they ask general questions, rather than asking specifics such as 'Is it Mr Mac?'

One rule is that the first question asked must not be 'Is it a man?' or 'Is it a woman?' (as this discounts a whole category too quickly). You can ask that after your opponent has asked their first question.

Once you get down to just two pictures you can guess a person.

Extra refinements

When choosing pictures for the game it is a good plan to have roughly equal numbers of pictures of males and females. For ease of play it's also a good idea to choose the photos with the most individual features: glasses, hats, scarves, beetling eyebrows, or indeed beards, are good news! However, if your staff all look a bit similar you can modify the question-asking part to include topics such as type of job; such as 'Does this person work in the office?' or 'Do they work in the kitchen?'

Variations

Alternatively, you could use pictures of celebrities if you feel that your clients have already learnd the names of staff.

The game can be adapted for team play, but make sure that everyone takes a turn.

Face-out descriptions

This is a simple, early approach to helping people remember and describe each other. It is suitable for a group of less able clients, or young children.

Materials

No materials are required, but all clients need to be sitting on chairs at a table. The seating should be arranged in such a way that the clients face each other, and include yourself at the table.

Procedure

Step 1: start with yourself. Look carefully at the person opposite and describe them, and encourage them to describe you. Then each client follows, describing the person opposite. This gives a general idea about which sorts of things to point out. (I remember a talk by Tony Attwood in which he mentioned one of his clients describing another person as having 'lovely red gums'!) Make a point of talking about the key features – beard or not, glasses or not, colour of hair, colour and type of clothing are examples.

Step 2: clients on one side of the table change places so that they are all opposite someone new.

Step 3: the new opposite partners take a look at each other, remembering the point about key features, then everyone on both sides of the table turns their chairs round, to face away from their partner. Now, in turns, they describe their partner, without, of course, peeping round to see!

Step 4: at the next session repeat step 3 only, that is, missing out the preparatory looking task, to see whether the principles of what to look for and how to remember what a person looks like have been established.

Speechmark

Friendship bands

This is a good way to bond a group of children or teenagers, promoting trust between them. They will be proud of the finished, personalised article, which will partly have been made by other group members, so the social skills of giving and receiving are also practised. Girls are really keen on these items, but boys are usually fine with them too. This method is an adaptation of the complex knotted variety.

You might occasionally have in your group a client who feels the need to sabotage the activity by writing inappropriate things. You will need to sit by this client and help them to see the benefits of being more positive, or help them by doing their part of the writing for them.

Materials needed

- Narrow white cotton tape (the narrowest you can find).
- Thick, soft (but not hairy) wool in many colours.
- Red and black biros (or other colours to suit).
- Scissors.
- String.

Getting started

The clients need to choose their four favourite colours of wool and cut off lengths of about 50cm. They also need the same length of white cotton tape.

They write their own name in red biro at one end of the tape. Now – this is the bit about trusting potential friends – they pass their tape around the group for others to add, in black biro, their compliments about the named person. Compliments might include such things as 'Nice hair', 'Has a good sense of humour' and 'Good at sharing'. The writers should also add their names. The superior version repeats this process on the other side of the tape, because as the band is made the tape will tend to fold in on itself, partly hiding some of the writing.

Now the band is given back to the owner. You may like to use this opportunity to encourage the clients to practise their presenting and receiving skills, maybe slightly exaggerating the 'thank you's' for the compliments.

Procedure

The band is formed by plaiting, using the tape as one of the three components, and two pairs of wool lengths for the other parts. A loop is needed at one end of the band – to form one half of the fastening when the band is worn – so tie this in very firmly at the beginning, poke some string through the loop, and use this to attach that end to the back of a chair, so making the plaiting process much easier. Plait the three components together, stopping short of the end.

Some of the clients may have no idea of how to plait, and clients with dyspraxia may find it quite difficult, but my advice is to let them do it themselves, taking their time over it, and give a little help here and there if you can see a potential fashion disaster forming! If they find the plaiting really too difficult, another method would be to twist the lengths together tightly, so that they will double back on themselves and hold when the lengths are folded in half (but you will need longer strings for that version).

Untie the string at the end of the band to free it from the chair, and measure around the wearer's wrist. Make a knot at the end of the wrist measurement, and another one at the end of the whole thing, leaving a fringe at the end.

You should now have the following formation on each band: a loop – a knot – a length of plait or twist that fits round the wrist – another knot – a free length of wools and tape – another knot – and a fringe.

To wear the band you push the fringe and free lengths through the loop, and tie off gently, using a knot that can easily be undone. Each client now has a personalised band, with compliments and the names of all group members on it, so they will find it easier to remember everyone's names.

Gift list

This is an 'awareness of others' game, useful any time, but particularly appropriate for therapy sessions leading up to Christmas, or festivals connected with other cultures. The idea is to try to think of gifts that would be appropriate for a range of people with different backgrounds. It can be done as an individual task but is more fun and often more productive as a group exercise. It is useful for learning to appreciate other people's interests and preferences, and can help with conversation techniques and friendship building. It can also be used as a real way of preparing for Christmas.

Materials needed

- Semi-official-looking forms. You could either make them yourself, photocopy the partially filled-in example overleaf, or use the blank grid and add other examples of people types as appropriate. If clients want to make real present buying lists they will need the names of the actual recipients down the side.

- At a pinch you could manage without the forms altogether if you've no time to prepare them; in which case you would just make lists.

- Pens.

- Also – but not essential – shopping catalogues for suggestions if clients are stuck for ideas.

Procedure

No matter what the ability level of your group, it would be wise to begin by discussing the list and together filling in a set of ideas for one type of person. Try to include in your discussions such topics as: how to find out what other people like; how to manage a present-buying budget; other occasions where presents are given; things you can make rather than buy.

You could add price limits for each of the gift levels mentioned – (1) pocket money gifts, (2) slightly more expensive offerings, and (3) something really luxurious, pretending you are very rich.

The clients might like to work in pairs, which will offer an opportunity for them to discuss and try to agree on ideas. If they prefer to work individually they can share the ideas after they have finished making their lists.

Gift list

Type of person	Modest gift	More expensive gift	Really expensive gift
A friend who is keen on sport			
An elderly grandma or grandad who likes gardening and going for country walks			
A six-year-old girl			
A ten-year-old boy			
A friend who is the same age as you and has similar interests			
A teenager who loves clothes			
A friend who is keen on art			
A businessperson who is 'stressed out'			
Someone who is home all day with young children			
A baby			

Speechmark

Gift list

Type of person	Modest gift	More expensive gift	Really expensive gift

Speechmark ⑤ 31

Haven't you changed!

A series of games to encourage observation of other people. It is a good opportunity, also, to practise sign language. It is designed for a small group of clients.

Materials needed

- Scarves.

- Hats.

- Glasses or shades.

- Ribbons.

- Hairbands.

- Jackets.

- Joke shop red noses.

- Glasses with built-in noses.

- Spock ears.

- and so on.

Procedure

There are several, progressively harder, ways to approach this.

In version 1, you must have the change items outside the room. One of the clients is scrutinised by the others, goes out, puts on a hat or a pair of glasses, or removes their cardigan or bangle, then returns to the room, and the others say what has changed.

In version 2, a client goes out of the room, while someone left *inside* changes something about themselves, for example, puts on a jacket, with the others in the group remaining neutral. The other client returns and examines those who remained in the room, selecting the 'changer'.

In version 3, a client goes out of the room and the others decide on a facial expression, a Makaton sign or a way of sitting, for example, arms or legs crossed. They are all adopting this expression or doing this action when the client returns for a short while to look at them, but nothing is said. Now the client goes out again, and the group adopts a different facial expression, Makaton sign or pose, and on coming back in the client must state what is different about the group.

A still more difficult version 4 is a new take on a well-tried parlour game. One person exits, and the others decide on an overt action and a covert action. The overt action could be to pass round, for example, an open or closed book, but covertly the action is sitting with the legs either apart or together. When the person re-enters the room they sit down with the

Speechmark

group and try to join in with the group's activity. The first one in the group (one who is 'in on' the secret) states 'I pass on this book open', or, 'I pass on this book closed'. The book will be randomly open or closed; it is the position of the legs that goes with the words. The one who is excluded from the secret tries to work out what the covert posture is.

Another statement could be 'I pass on these scissors crossed', or 'I pass on these scissors uncrossed'; again, that would happen randomly while it would be the legs that were crossed or uncrossed. You could try 'I pass on this tea towel folded' or 'I pass on this tea towel unfolded', when it would actually be the arms that were folded or not. (Passing the towel on with folded arms is possible to do!) Or try 'I pass on this pencil upright' or 'I pass on this pencil leaning', but it would really be your posture that was upright, or inclining slightly to one side. Then there could be 'I pass on this pen pointing up' or 'I pass on this pen pointing down', and with the other hand slightly pointing up or down. Your own or your clients' imaginations will suggest more of these; all you have to remember is that you need a statement which can apply both to an object and to a bodily action.

Road sign dominoes

This game promotes careful observation, road safety, and conversation about road manners (a form of self- or other awareness!). It is useful for clients who have grown out of picture dominoes, but who find the traditional black-and-white dots game boring. It is also useful for those who are current or potential drivers. You can also use it to promote the skill of careful looking. It is designed to be a group activity.

Materials needed

- You need to obtain at least two Highway Codes. In fact, four would be better, as then you can use both sides of each page. You need two of each picture. If you have access to a colour photocopier you can cut costs by copying images from just one Highway Code.

- Good quality card, or 'Taskmaster' blank cards. My advice is not to scrimp on this, as you need to present your (quite expensive) pictures in the best possible way.

- Glue.

- Scissors.

Making the dominoes

Cut out the road signs and keep them together in their pairs. Bear in mind that each card will need to show two different signs. You will need to line up the cards and stick one of each pair of signs on the touching sides of adjacent cards. The first half of the first card will match up with the last half of the last card.

Procedure

Play as for other forms of dominoes.

Discuss why we have rules of the road, and make the point that politeness on the road, for example, allowing another driver to go ahead in front of you, not 'cutting in' on another car, and so on, can prevent accidents and road rage. Mention that this kind of courtesy is very much liked by other drivers. Also discuss the links between polite driving and the way that we behave when we are not inside our cars, for example, how we use pavement space, how we queue or how close we stand to the person in front at the checkout.

Variations

Stick pairs of pictures on different cards, and use for a Snap game, or as a variation of Pelmanism, the memory game described in the 'Car logo Pelmanism' game in Chapter 8 'Memory'.

Standing in your shoes

The idea of this activity is to help the clients to become more aware and tolerant of other people's ideas and perspectives. It is carried out in pairs, perhaps partnering established friends, or maybe less well-acquainted people. It also promotes interviewing skills. It is quite an intimate activity, involving touch and possibly smell! In my experience, if you approach it light-heartedly there will not be complaints. There is also the possibility of introducing some work on related figurative language at some point during the session.

Materials needed

- Large pieces of paper – we found that halved flipchart sheets were fine.

- Water-based wide felt tip pens for the outline drawing; narrow ones for the writing.

Procedure

In pairs, draw around each other's shoes. It is easier to do this with the shoes off, but make sure that the clients are not drawing round their own shoes – it's important that they find out about their partner. Make sure they do not draw on the shoes, especially if the shoes are a pale colour, and be sure to use felt tips that are water based and washable.

Now one of the partners asks the other one questions on how the partner feels about all sorts of subjects and why. They then write their name and opinions in the shoe outlines. For example, 'I prefer to borrow movies on DVDs rather than go to the cinema because I don't like such a loud noise', or 'I am a vegetarian because I once saw a TV programme about abattoirs', or 'I'm against pedestrian zones because they are scary at night'. Try to fit in as many comments as possible. Now swap over and let the other partner do the interviewing and writing.

Conclude the session by having a discussion about the expression 'standing in your shoes' and how it is possible to tolerate other people's ideas once you know why they feel as they do.

Compare the saying 'standing in your shoes', with 'seeing it from your perspective', 'on the same wavelength', 'singing from the same hymn sheet (or song sheet)' and any other connected sayings.

You might like to use these 'shoe sheets' as wall decorations.

Older or younger?

This game is based on the old favourite card game of 'Sevens'. This version promotes judgement of people's ages, which can be a very hard task for many clients, especially people on the autism spectrum, who may have no idea whether you are in your twenties or your sixties!

Ideally you will have four players, although you can play with three, five or six.

It is quite a complicated game to make and takes some time, but my advice is to take a deep breath and go for it. It will prove to be a useful resource.

Materials needed

- Twenty-eight blank cards – the 'Taskmaster' ones are good (but quite small), or you can use blank business cards, index cards, postcards, or even unwanted playing cards if you can find large enough photos of people to cover the original faces of the cards. (However, if you use these you might as well take advantage of them by leaving a corner of the original card on view showing which suit that card belongs to.)

- PVA glue.

- Stick-on stars.

- Pen.

- Lined paper.

- Magazines.

- Paperclips.

Procedure

Cut out magazine pictures of people of varying ages and backgrounds. You need to have four sets of seven cards that range in age. You need four babies, four toddlers, four children, four teenagers, four young adults, four middle-aged people and four older people. They need to be able to fit on the cards, and within each set that ranges in age from babyhood to old age, there needs to be a vague resemblance, as if that baby could have grown into that older person (don't have a little girl growing into an old man, or a person changing to a different ethnicity!). Ideally you will have two sets of females and two of males. Try to find sets of photos depicting people from different ethnic backgrounds.

Good sources for pictures at the different stages are Mothercare catalogues, schoolwear catalogues, teen magazines, newspaper colour supplements and *Saga* magazines. Ideally the pictures should be of the whole body, but this is a counsel of perfection: you may have to compromise with head-and-shoulder shots.

Making the games

Plan the sticking of the pictures on to the cards by first just placing them, fastening them with a paperclip for now and sticking them on with glue later in the process.

Arrange the sets of cards into four vertical columns, with a baby at the bottom of each, then a toddler, then a child, and so on until you have the four older people at the top of the columns.

To make clear the separate sets, you can edge each card within a set with a colour, so you would make seven blue-edged ones ranging from babyhood to old age, seven orange, and so on. If you use real playing cards you could arrange each of your sets on one playing card suit – hearts, clubs, spades, diamonds – leaving a corner of the original card visible, to show which cards go together.

Now number the cards, writing in the top right-hand corner of each card as follows: babies are 1, toddlers are 2, children are 3, teenagers are 4, young adults are 5, middle-aged people are 6 and older people are 7. Stick stars by the teenagers.

Playing the 'Older or younger?' game

Deal out five cards each (more players = fewer cards). Place the spare cards face down on the table as the 'stack'. The rules are the same as for ordinary 'Sevens'. If you are not familiar with this game it may look complicated, but actually it is very easy. These are the rules:

The player to the left of the dealer picks up a card from the stack, adding it to their hand. They then put down, face up, a 'teenager' (the starred card), if they have one. If they have not got a 'teenager' they discard one card (to the bottom of the stack), and play passes to their left. This continues until a player gets a teenager card, which is placed face up, with the play then passing to the left.

After a 'teenager' card has been put down the next player takes a card from the stack, and then either puts down another teenager face up next to the first teenager, or puts a slightly older or younger person if the same suit above or below the teenager card, that is, the numbers will be consecutive. They then discard a card.

Play then passes to their left. This player can add another teenager card next to the existing teenager cards, or add a card above or below any of the cards currently displayed, providing of course that the card placed down is in the right chronological sequence and of the same suit. You should end up with four lines of people cards ranging in age, with three people cards below the teenager leading back to babyhood, and three above leading to old age. The one who is first to use all of their cards is the winner.

Discuss with the group the changes that often take place in people's appearance as they age, covering such topics as ability to walk, growth in height, growth of facial hair, even wrinkles, greying hair and postural decline (if not too depressing!). You might want to be prepared that some clients will be very interested in the changes that take place at puberty. If you don't feel able to discuss this in the SLT setting then you will need to engineer things to avoid that topic, or say, 'we won't discuss that now, but you could talk about it with your teacher'. I've found, however, that if you are just straightforward and answer the questions they ask, you will find that it is all they need.

Variations

Use the same cards, but simply place the cards in age order. This is an easier activity which still demonstrates the ageing process.

For a superior version, add two more sets of cards. This will further emphasise the way that people age, and means that the game will last longer. If you've used playing cards as the bases you'll have to apply sticker shapes on the extra sets.

As with any activity, you can use some of the discussion time to include related vocabulary, and colloquial or idiomatic language. So, for example, here you could discuss: ' …hood' (eg babyhood, boyhood); 'silver surfers'; 'OAPs'; 'salad days'; 'to come of age'; 'key of the door'; 'an awkward age' and 'ripe old age'. If the group seems willing they might like to discuss ageism as a connected topic.

Tourist information game

This is another 'awareness of others' game, very closely linked to 'Gift list'. It follows the same pattern but is more relevant to other times of the year. The idea is to try to think of appropriate outings for people with different backgrounds. The game aims to stimulate ideas about other people's interests and preferences, and can also be a way of planning real days out, for friendship building.

Materials needed

- Semi-official-looking forms. You could either make them yourself, or photocopy the partially filled-in example overleaf, or use the blank grid and add other examples of people types as appropriate.

- Alternatively you could manage without the forms altogether, if you've no time to prepare them, in which case you would just make lists.

- Some clients may need to have photos to enhance their understanding of the character types. These could be found in magazines or colour supplements.

- The game is very much enhanced if you have leaflets and brochures about places to visit, if you have the time to go and collect them (you can get these from real tourist information centres or visitor information centres.) For some groups you might also add a map.

- Pens.

Carrying out the activity

No matter what the ability level of your group, it would be wise to begin by discussing the list and together filling in a set of ideas for their day out, for one type of person.

Try to include in your discussions such topics as:

- How to find out what other people would like to do, bearing in mind the advantages and disadvantages of keeping it a secret versus surprising them.

- How to manage transport for the day.

- How capable they are, for instance, would an elderly person or someone on crutches manage a walk, or would a young child cope with a long day out?

- How often might they need to stop?

- The budget – who pays? Are there places where you might go that are cheap or free?

The clients might like to work in pairs, which will offer an opportunity for them to discuss and try to agree on ideas. If they prefer to work individually they can share the ideas after they have finished making their lists.

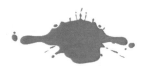

Tourist information game

Type of person	Morning	Lunch	Afternoon and evening
A sporty friend who is on crutches due to a sprained ankle			
A six-year-old girl			
A ten-year-old boy			
A man who likes fishing			
An older lady who likes music			
A gourmet (someone who just loves food!)			
A teenage Goth			
A businessperson or woman who is 'stressed out'			
A teacher			
A friend who needs cheering up			

Tourist information game

Type of person	Morning	Lunch	Afternoon and evening

Timeline

This activity helps students to learn about time, people's ages and history.

You will need to place this piece of work on a long wall, so bear in mind that the length of the paper will depend on whether you think your timeline will turn out to be small, neat and tidy, or big and sprawling, maybe with illustrations. It will also depend on how long a period of time you want to represent. Also remember that when your group of students finds out how very old you are, you will be the subject of much mirth. My advice is to make sure some other, even older, members of staff are mentioned on it or some old celebrities who are rated as 'cool', for example, football coaches, or movie or TV characters!

Materials needed

- Long roll of paper – we used craft paper sold this way, but you could use decorators' lining paper.
- Felt tip pens.
- Photos.
- Magazines.

Procedure

Decide how long you want your timeline to represent. We began just before the Second World War, but you may have some fossil fanatics in your group who would want prehistoric times included.

Draw a line centrally, the length of the paper, and divide this line into one-, ten- and hundred-year sections (if you include prehistory you'll have to have thousand- and million-year sections, perhaps in a different colour which would allow you to represent them in an abbreviated form.)

Mark on it some important events – some connected with world events, some with politics, some with sport, some with royalty, some with the emergence or break-up of pop bands, and whatever else is a popular topic in your group. You might include the founding date of your school or college.

Together, write on your chart the dates of birth of people in your organisation, and of your group members and maybe, if appropriate, of their parents and grandparents. Count up the sections from their birth date to the present day to show how being born earlier means you will be older. You can now talk about concepts of time and look at magazine, newspaper or other photos to demonstrate how people age.

If your group includes artists, you could illustrate your timeline, or you could add photos or magazine pictures.

Other ideas for raising awareness of others

Please see also:

1 '"Same and different chains"', in Chapter 2 'Self-awareness and self-esteem'.

2 'Fields of interest' in Chapter 15 'Wallcharts and decorations'.

3 'Interaction paper chains for Christmas' in Chapter 15 'Wallcharts and decorations'.

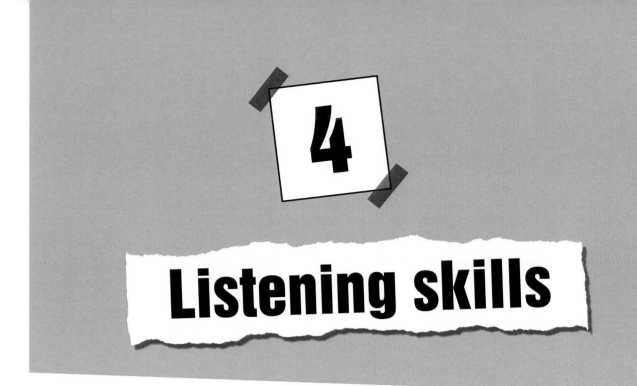

4

Listening skills

Have you ever tried listening to somebody talking to you when there is a great deal of background noise? Or looking politely interested when you are far more fascinated by the conversation at the next table in the café? Or focusing fully on a lecture or 'worthy' TV programme when you would really rather be doing something else?

A good test of your own ability to focus, listen, discriminate between competing sounds, and remember, is to turn on the weather forecast (no, not the very brief version!), and at the end attempt to recall the information that was given, not just for your own geographical region, but also for other areas of the country. Unless you are unusually well focused I suspect that you will find this a fairly difficult challenge. Now try to recall that information after an hour or so has passed. Now try remembering it again with another sound going on, maybe a piece of music, or a play on the radio. These represent various challenges to our ability to listen effectively.

Imagine experiencing one or more of those challenges all the time, but with the added problems of having to ask for repetition, and of coping with the irritation of others when they need to repeat several times.

This next comment is not intended to be 'preachy' (if you find it that way then please move on to the fun bit – the activities), but a key way to help with listening skills is to request all those who work or associate with the client to adopt careful strategies to help your client listen and remember what has been said.

These strategies would include some or all of the following, that is, staff should:

- make sure they can be heard – keep any competing background noise down; speak clearly; face the client with the light shining towards the speaker rather than the client

- break their talk into short chunks, observing or questioning to make sure that the client has understood

- be brief – overloading the client with information is often the main obstruction to listening to the whole message

- be interesting and humorous or light-hearted, but clear.

The games and activities in this chapter aim to help with listening in general, and to focus particularly on auditory discrimination and auditory memory.

Sound effects

This is an excellent and funny listening game for a group of older children or young teenagers. They will be learning to listen very carefully for the right moment to chip in with the appropriate sound.

Materials needed

A few short pre-written stories that would be enhanced by sound effects. These can be your own stories, or could be taken from a book.

Procedure

Read the story aloud to the group, just going straight through it without stopping. Now go back over it and discuss potential sound effects that could be added. Retell the story, leaving small gaps to be filled by the clients making the appropriate noises. They will need to listen very carefully and be prepared to 'chip in' with the appropriate sound as soon as they hear the cue.

Example

One windy day (*wind – howling noise*) we went for a walk on a farm, squelching through deep mud (*squelching noise*). We were laughing with each other (*laugh*) and enjoying the sounds of the farm animals (*various farm animal noises*) when all of a sudden we heard the most tremendous crash (*crashing noise*).

Across the field we saw that a barn had begun to collapse, and beams were still thudding down (*thuds*). We ran across there as quickly as we could in the squelching mud (*fast squelching sounds*) to see if anyone needed help.

Under the collapsed roof we could hear someone calling (*Help! Help!*) and we wondered what to do (*What shall we do? What shall we do?*). We rang the fire brigade from my mobile (*ringing, requesting help*) and in the meantime tried reassuring the trapped person that help was on its way. It seemed to soothe the person – who turned out to be a boy called Tom – to whistle pop songs to him (*whistle a pop song*).

Soon the fire engine and an ambulance arrived, sirens blaring (*siren noises*) and the firefighter moved the heavy beams with a great effort (*sounds of effortful straining*). Tom was not badly hurt, mostly just frightened, but as he was lifted out he remembered his dog Buster who was lost, and who might also be under the collapsed roof. We told him that the firefighter would look for the dog and that we would help. Off Tom went in the ambulance (*siren*). We called and called for Buster (*Buster, Buster*), who eventually came bounding up to us from another field, barking loudly (*woof, woof*). We looked after Buster for a few days, until Tom was out of hospital, and then the two were reunited, very pleased to see each other, with Tom laughing and the dog barking (*woofing and laughing*).

If the clients enjoyed this game they might like to try writing their own story that could undergo the same treatment, for all to enjoy. Write the stories down and copy them into a small book that the clients could keep, to think about at other times, or perhaps for them to try at home with their families.

Noises off

Many of our clients, especially those with auditory processing difficulties, find it difficult to listen to speech because they are distracted by background noise, or their ears may hear sounds in an unequal way. This exercise aims to help them practise discriminating between the wanted sounds of talking and any unwanted noise.

Here is an individual exercise and a group version.

Materials needed

- Recordings of various songs, music, people chatting, traffic noise and white noise (white noise is obtainable from the radio – slightly tune it out or off the station and you will get a hissing sound).

- A magazine of the client's choice.

Procedure

Play white noise fairly quietly, and while it plays read just a few words from a magazine. Ask them to tell you what you said. You need to be sure that your chosen sentence or phrase is not too long, otherwise you will be working with auditory memory rather than or as well as auditory discrimination.

If they can manage to pick out what you have said, then go on to a slightly harder discrimination exercise, with louder white noise but keeping your voice at the same volume level as before. Build up gradually over several sessions using progressively louder, more complex and more attractive background sounds, playing the recordings of songs, traffic, chattering, and so on, but with your voice remaining not too loud. Try to avoid a situation where they fail.

In a group setting you can divide the clients into two teams, with one group listening and the other group humming, singing, whispering or chatting at various volume levels while you ask a question or give a short message or instruction for the listeners to act on. Your question could be something like 'What day is it?', or the instruction could be 'Scratch your ear'.

Market traders

Have you ever been in an old-fashioned street market where the stallholders shout out to entice you to look at their wares? Sometimes several shout at the same time, which makes for an interesting mix of sounds. This fun game, based on that type of sound mix, is for a fairly large group, ideally eight to ten participants. It calls for careful listening skills, and teamwork. A basic knowledge of syllable splitting is also useful. The idea is that everyone in one team will shout out a different syllable all at the same time, and the other team has to work out what they are shouting.

Materials needed

- Copy of the week's TV listings.

- List of the current top 20 pop songs in the charts (*Top of the Pops* magazine is excellent for this, or you can find out online).

- List of films.

- List of pop singers.

- List of sportspeople.

Procedure

As a whole group, decide whether you are going to shout out names of pop songs, singers, TV programmes or films. To avoid confusion, put the unwanted lists away, leaving out just one list, let's say films.

Divide into two subgroups, A and B, and instruct each team to choose a leader.

Each group chooses something from the list – for example, group A might choose *The King's Speech*. (This title is a good one for a group of three as it has three single-syllable words.) Choosing the title and practising the simultaneous shout needs to be done out of earshot of the opposing team (or very quietly). Each person in group A is assigned a word. When group B is ready and listening, and at a signal from their leader, group A shout out their words *all at the same time*, so that what is heard is one multilayered sound.

Now, group B must work out what was said.

They then take a turn, but this time, suppose they have chosen *Titanic*. Now each member of group B must be given one *syllable* to shout simultaneously.

You may find that you cannot find a film with the right number of syllables in the title, so then you will have to get one person to say two syllables at double speed, or maybe one syllable very slowly.

Variation

The original party version of this game uses proverbs, and this is excellent if your clients are already aware of these sayings, or if you would like to promote more use of such figurative language.

Rally navigator

This is good for listening skills, concentration, organising and prioritising sentences, and incidentally for getting to know the locality. Participants will need to know their left and right.

Materials needed

- A large-scale map (or part of one) of the local area, photocopied (perhaps enlarged) for each group member.

- Pencils, paper and envelope.

Procedure

Take it in turns to be the 'navigator', but it's probably best if you go first, so that you can convey the general idea.

Decide on the destination, and secretly write it down on paper, which is then placed in the envelope. State the starting point (eg a school) and have in mind a route towards the secret end point. Make sure that everyone has their finger on the start, and begins by going the right way.

Now simply direct the group members to turn left or right at various landmarks en route to the destination.

Asking for clarification is to be encouraged as a skill. Depending on the ability level of the group they can try to make the questions as verbal as possible, or can be allowed some visual clues.

When someone reaches the correct point and calls out to say so, you can congratulate them and show the paper in the envelope to prove that you have not changed the destination.

Now the play passes either to that winner or to the person on your left. They think of a new destination, write it down and place it in the envelope as before, and state the new starting point.

The exercise is even more worthwhile if the clients cannot see one another's progress, because otherwise they may just copy each other; however, the downside of that is that they may worry about failure, so you will have to be sensitive to their needs.

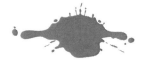

Soap box

This is a listening, remembering, understanding and analysing activity which can be applied to conversational technique, especially length of turn or contribution. Because it uses popular radio and TV programmes, there is usually no trouble motivating clients to do this work. Many clients on the autism spectrum find that they can learn useful tips about chatting to people from TV conversations, because they can observe in a detached way, without having to make eye contact. This activity works well for a group of four or five teenagers, or you could use it one-to-one with an adult client.

Materials needed

- Recordings of radio or TV soaps, such as *The Archers*, *EastEnders* or *Coronation Street*. Use whichever programme is deemed to be 'cool'. Record a longish piece of conversation in which two or three people are talking pleasantly and evenly – not arguing. You will, of course, need the right equipment in your clinic to play it back.

- Paper and pens.

- Stopwatch.

Procedure

Introduce the recording carefully, setting the conversation in its context.

Ask one client to time the conversational turns and another to write this data down. Listen to or watch the piece, jotting down the turn timings. You will probably find, as we did, that most conversational turns in soaps last for about four to six seconds. This can be quite a revelation for the conversational 'ramblers'! If you feel it to be appropriate for your group you could then time the length of the real conversational turns in your session.

Variations

You can use this method for examining other aspects of conversation, for example, eye contact, facial expression or topic choice. You may be able to find pieces of the programme that illustrate friendship skills, for example, compromising on what to do, letting the friend go first, telling the truth or offering a compliment.

Be careful to analyse for only one skill at a time.

Sometimes I find myself working with a group of 'telly addicts' who are so interested in the medium that they have few or no other interests to talk about. If this happens you could try demonstrating one small aspect of TV that is designed to keep our eyes on the screen, such as fast cutting from one image to another. Simply ask the clients to say each time they notice when the image cuts to another. They will soon see how often this happens, and once they understand how the programme makers think, they may become more discerning and begin to think of alternative leisure activities.

Which service do you require?

Making a toy telephone is an activity to promote speaking and listening. It is fun to make and use, and gives practical guidance about how to telephone the emergency services.

You need, ideally, to have the use of a long corridor, or two rooms opposite each other, with doors that could be nearly closed (but beware of tripping or garrotting or otherwise wounding passers-by!)

Materials needed

- Two empty metal cans, or cylindrical cardboard containers with metal bases, such as those used for powdered milk.

- A long piece of string or cord, say 10m.

- Sticky tape.

- If possible, two bells or whistles.

Procedure

Make any sharp metal edges safe by sticking tape over them.

In the centre of the base of each can, make a hole that is just large enough to thread the string through.

Ask two clients to stand as far apart as possible so that the string is taut.

To start with, each client tests the system by saying something in a normal voice, and then using progressively quieter volume, until the other client cannot hear them through the air, only through the 'telephone'.

Now practise 'making a call'. To do this, one client takes on the role of the 'operator', while the other is the person in need of help.

The operator is alerted when they hear the bell. They will need to say 'Which service do you require?' and the caller will name police, fire or ambulance. The operator will also ask about the caller's location and for a few details about the problem.

The clients then switch roles.

Variations

You can use this method for other types of phone conversations, for example, making arrangements to meet and go out together, passing on information or just having a chat.

Other ideas to help with listening skills

Please see also:

1 'Talking stick', in Chapter 5 'Conversation skills'.

2 'My news and yours', also in Chapter 5 'Conversation skills'.

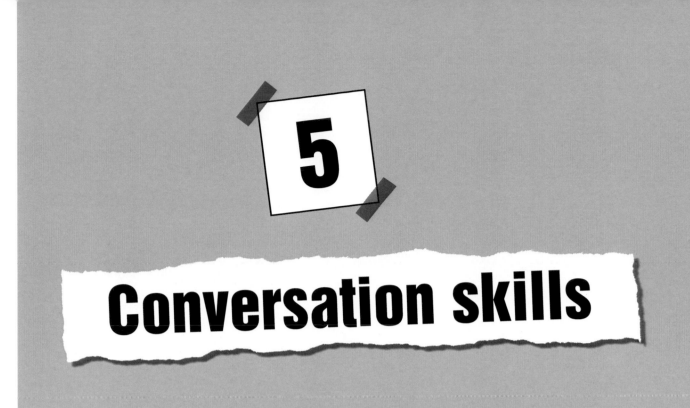

Conversation skills

What is a conversation? Defining what we mean by 'conversation' is quite a difficult task because it takes many different forms: the quick chat on the way to work or in a shop; the friendly short or long phone call; the extended conversation where intimacies are shared; the complex exchange of compliments, opinions, jokes and sympathetic comments at a dinner party, and so on. Even interviews are a kind of formalised conversation, but with special rules.

For many of our clients it is very difficult indeed to decipher the 'codes' of conversational styles that are appropriate in any given setting.

Some interesting research by BT (reported in a paper at the Market Research Society Conference 1995) looked at British views of phone conversations, partly for the purpose of developing its advertising campaigns.

In this piece of research some participants defined 'big talk', as 'important, male, serious, official, correct'. On the other hand, 'small talk' was considered by some to be 'unimportant, female, trivial, popular, incorrect'.

However, the researchers also found that although small talk is often belittled as prattle, idle gossip, tittle-tattle and so on, it has an important role in our lives as a form of 'social knitting', that is, binding together families and communities, whereas 'big talk' is more to do with business activities.

Many clients with a diagnosis on the autism spectrum are much more at ease with 'big talk' than small talk, but in fact they need to improve their small talk skills if they aim to converse well in social settings, and it is small talk which is the main focus of this chapter.

Some of the activities here would be referred to as 'narrative skills' by speech and language therapists. These are the kinds of speaking which rely on the client's ability to report, tell or retell, in an appropriately prioritised and well-sequenced way.

Talking stick

This is a useful, cheap and easy item to make with a teenage social language group where taking turns seems to be a problem, either because they are overly keen to get their point in, or because they are reluctant to take up a turn. It will help if the group is already interested in Native American people and their culture – maybe linking with a classroom project – but this is not absolutely vital and you yourself may be able to enthuse them about the culture by showing pictures or books about the Native American culture.

Materials needed

- You need a stick. I would tend to err on the side of 'too small' rather than 'too big', as sticks can be used as weapons! Also, if it is smallish you will be able to store it in a cardboard tube (eg one from a roll of kitchen paper).

- String.

- Scissors and glue.

- Beads – nice wooden ones or small glass ones would add to the quality of and respect for this item, which you may find yourself using in such groups for years.

- A few feathers.

Making the talking stick

Make a groove round the stick, using a penknife – probably best to do this bit on your own before the session, to avoid disaster!

Tie the string round the stick, and attach the beads and feathers to the string.

Procedure

It will be helpful to have a list of discussion subjects relevant to your particular client group. These could be local or national newspaper headlines, or issues currently topical to the school or college where you work (they could be to do with clothes, food, etc). Try to make the subject something that they have opinions about.

Each group member should be encouraged to offer an opinion, but may only speak while they are holding the stick. Begin by passing the stick in order round the circle, but work towards a freer form, where group members silently indicate their desire to speak, so producing a more natural conversation. If you have an 'over-wordy' person in the group you may need to introduce a half-minute rule, so that the others do not get bored. Take care to arrange it so that reluctant speakers also join in.

It is worth remembering that turn taking not only requires the disciplines of joining in and waiting for a turn, but also of remembering what you have to say until a good moment arrives.

Before doing this activity it may be useful, as I have found, to allow a group to talk all at once and then point out that the conversation is not working because no one can hear what anyone else is saying. Then you will have good grounds for proceeding.

Variation

You could use a real or fake microphone instead of the talking stick. My preference would still be for the stick, as it places the emphasis on conversation and turn taking, rather than on performing, which would tend to go with the microphone idea.

Speechmark

DIY ball

If clients make their own materials they value them more, and will tend to remember the activity associated with the item. Ball games are useful for establishing better turn taking. This activity links to the previous one, 'Talking stick'.

Materials needed

- Strong round balloons in many colours (three for each participant).
- Dried lentils.
- Funnel.
- Trays (one for each participant).

Making the DIY ball

Each client does the following:

Take one balloon and, working over the tray, fill it with lentils using the funnel. Aim for a size a bit bigger than a ping-pong ball, but not as big as a tennis ball.

Once you have the required size, tie the balloon off. Leaving a short length to avoid the knot coming undone, cut off the thick rim part of the balloon tie. Now you have the basic ball shape.

Take a second balloon in a different colour, and cut off the very end of the knot area. Cut a few (three or four) small round holes in this balloon, and pull it on to the basic ball, covering the knot in the first balloon, and allowing the colour of the balloon underneath to show through. You will not have to knot this balloon.

Now repeat this procedure using a third colour of balloon, and the clients will have a handmade multicoloured ball showing areas of all the colours.

Note: it is possible to stuff the first balloon with cottonwool balls or polystyrene bobbles instead, if your group needs a lightweight alternative.

Using the balls

The rule for taking turns is that only the person with the ball is allowed to speak, so first of all you need to place all the newly made balls in a bowl on the table to avoid confusion. Now take one of the balls, and have a round of 'My favourite film is …', passing the ball on after each person has stated their preference. Then you could have a round of 'My favourite weekend activity is …' using another ball, and so on until everyone has had a chance to use their own creation as a therapy tool.

Balls can also be used in a name-learning game. Each participant says their name, then, once they seem to be remembering each other's names, take turns to say your name followed by the name of the person to whom you are throwing the ball, then that person says their name and the name of another participant, and so on.

Question dice

Useful in group sessions for conversation building and to practise question formation.

Materials needed

- Upholsterer's foam 10cm-deep – safer than wood!

- Indelible ink pen.

Brawn needed

Cut the foam into 10cm cubes. Some upholsterers will cut the sponge for you but, if not, it's easiest to cut it with a bread knife.

Suggestion: make several, as these sorts of cubes are useful for other activities too.

Completing the cubes

On each face of one of the dice, write one of these question beginners: Who, What, Where, When, Why and How. (You could write other word classes, such as adverbs or conjunctions, on the other cubes, to use in other games.)

Procedure

Take turns to roll the dice and ask another member of the group a question beginning with the word on the face of the dice. The client who is answering should give a brief response and then take their turn at asking someone else a question.

You could develop this – as I do – by presenting alongside photo cards of people doing various occupations or activities, and pretend that they are actually present in the group and think up questions to ask them. Discuss the possible responses. I also have a silver inflatable 'alien' who sometimes sits in the group and is asked questions – the group has to think what the response would be!

Further use

The question dice are also useful for sign language practice on staff training days.

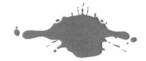

Just a minute

This is an activity for a group of fairly able clients who tend to go off topic, or generally lose focus, or leave long pauses in their discourse. The name of the game is not meant to indicate that a minute is the right length for a normal conversational turn (in fact, it is usually too long), but rather that if they are ever asked to talk about their weekend, or holiday, say, they will not be fazed by the task. They need to already be familiar with the ideas of prioritising and organising what they are going to say. (Dr Wendy Rinaldi's *Language Choices* course is brilliant for this groundwork.)

You may feel that your group needs to work towards a shorter time, rather than begin with a minute — 30 or even 15 seconds may be a better starting point.

Materials needed

- Ideally, a recording of the excellent Radio 4 programme *Just a Minute*.
- Stopwatch.
- List of talk topics, numbered up to 20, and kept hidden.

Procedure

Listen to the recording, discussing the ideas about not hesitating, repeating or deviating from the subject. Remember that the speaker is allowed to repeat the words included in the title of the talk.

You should take the first turn, handing one of your clients the timer. Pick a number between 1 and 20, and talk about that numbered topic for the time decided. If you hesitate, deviate or repeat yourself, a client can knock on the table, the stopwatch is stopped, your fault is described and, if the challenge is allowed, the challenger takes up the topic and continues for the remainder of the time. Once your turn has been completed, you can be the 'chairman', as you may need to arbitrate from time to time.

If you decide to use a scoring system, the traditional arrangement is that you get a point for:

- speaking when the time is up
- making a correct challenge
- managing to keep going for a whole minute (or whatever time has been agreed)
- (at your discretion) making a humorous contribution.

Suggestions for topic list

1 A message in a bottle

2 Fire practice

3 How to spend £50

4 Jumble sales

5 Mobile phones

6 The most enjoyable day of the week

7 Fancy dress parties

8 My nicest surprise

9 A trip to the moon

10 Gardening

11 *Top of the Pops*

12 Holiday destinations

13 My favourite meal

14 The worst meal I ever had

15 Pets

16 Ice skating

17 Football

18 Cars

19 In 10 years

20 Shopping

It is probably best to avoid subjects that are obsessions or fascinations for any of the clients.

Folded paper fortune tellers

Do you remember making these at school? If not, your own or a neighbour's children may be able to help with folding the prototype. Fortune tellers promote making choices, encourage conversation, can be designed for different abilities, cost almost nothing and are good fun!

If you already know how to fold these things the first bit will seem very long-winded, so pass swiftly on to 'Completing'.

Materials needed

- Sheets of A3 paper, trimmed to a square. You need this larger size of paper so that you'll have enough room for all of the writing.

- Scissors and pens.

Folding the fortune teller

If you are managing a group on your own, a few trial runs beforehand would be a wise idea. It's easy really, though: you will soon be able to demonstrate making one at the same time as watching everybody else's progress.

It's best to do all the folding first, and then begin the writing in the areas formed.

Fold the square in half and then half again, to find the middle. Open it out so that you now have a flat piece of paper with a cross in the middle.

Fold the corners to the middle neatly, and flatten them down so that you now have a new, smaller sized square with folds along all of the outer edges and all the corner points meeting.

Turn the whole thing over so that the side with the corner points is face down. Now fold the newly formed corners to the middle as before.

Turn it over again and you'll see that you have made four little 'pockets' for your index finger and thumbs of each hand to poke into. Now pinch the whole thing together. This will be quite easy to do if you have done the folding neatly.

You should now have a three-dimensional object ready to write on. You will probably want to open it out a bit, to make the writing easier.

Completing

Now for the writing. On the outer four squares, formed on the back of the fortune teller (the part visible when you put your fingers into it), you will need to write the numbers 1 to 8 (one number each side of the fold on each square).

On the next part, the eight triangles within, you write four themes or situations, for example, 'Holiday Disasters', 'Nice Surprises', 'Lovely Foods and 'Wrong Clothes'. Place the 'desirable' themes opposite each other – in this way when the choosing part happens they will either have two nice or two nasty things to choose between. Now open the fortune teller up even more, to expose the inner part, and write three choices for each theme:

Holiday Disasters could include:

It will rain solidly for two days.

You will forget to bring your picnic on a day out.

The cinema will close due to a flood.

Nice Surprises could be:

You will find a five pound note in your pocket.

Some excellent musicians will perform in the street.

A beautiful butterfly will settle on your hand.

Lovely Foods might be:

You will have sausages and chips.

You will have crisps and a fizzy drink.

You will have a huge ice cream.

Wrong Clothes could include:

You have to wear a plastic bag hat because of the rain.

Your shoelace breaks, so you have to use hairy string.

You thought it was a casual party and put on old clothes, but everyone else is wearing smart gear.

The above is only an example; you can have whatever subjects enthuse your group. You might try a 'Talking situations' version, for instance:

The Waiting Room, with predictions such as:

The only other person there will think they know you.

You will be confronted by a beautiful girl (or boy).

Everyone will be sitting down and the only spare chair has a bag on it.

The Youth Club, with predictions such as:

The only activity available tonight will be table tennis, and you feel awkward trying that.

It will be disco night and all your favourite music will be played.

It will be snooker night but someone will have stolen the cues.

The School Reunion, with predictions such as:

The person who bullied you at school will be there.

Your favourite teacher will be delighted to see you.

A friend you lost touch with will come up and say hello.

The Birthday Party, with predictions such as:

There will be great fireworks at the end.

It will be a beach party and you will have a barbecue.

There will be good music and great food.

Once you have shown your examples of 'fortunes' written in this device, then you can encourage your clients to devise their own. Take care, though, that nothing too disastrous, offensive or rude is written.

Note: you can write eight situations if you can fit them on to the paper, and have enough ideas. You would then have to think of eight sets of choices.

How to use your fortune teller

One person pokes their fingers into their fortune teller and becomes the 'clairvoyant'. This person gives the instructions or asks the questions, while the other person, the 'fortune seeker', responds (which could be by pointing).

The first instruction is 'Choose a number between 1 and 8', and depending on the response the clairvoyant opens and closes the fortune teller that number of times, in opposite directions.

The next instruction is to choose between the situations revealed.

Once this is done ask the fortune seeker to pick a number between 1 and 3, and then the clairvoyant will read out the fortune.

Storyteller activity

The idea of this activity is to help the clients to improve their narrative skills. It is quite a challenge, but good fun for older teenagers.

Materials needed

- Magazine pictures of people doing different activities – the more varied the better.
- Words printed on cards.

These include 'story starters', for example, 'There was a sudden bang as my tyre went flat' or 'We had just won £100 so …' or 'We had run out of money while we were on holiday'.

Other cards would be 'atmospheric descriptors' such as 'The pub was full and the music played loudly' or 'It was a wintry night with snow swirling around the door' or 'The lake was peaceful'.

The third category of card would be 'story finishers' such as 'so eventually we were allowed to leave the café' or 'I was so pleased to get back home' or 'I will never go to that place again' or 'What would you have done?'

The fourth category of card gives single words or phrases graded to the ability of your client group. Easier ones could include 'lawnmower', 'fizzy pop', 'fridge' and while harder ones could include adjectives and adverbs such as 'cheerful', 'popular' and 'despondently'.

There are also 'random extras' such as nonsense words, for example, from Roald Dahl or Edward Lear – 'frobscottle', 'gimble', or you (or they) can invent some. For able groups, unusual or advanced vocabulary should also be included: for example, cookery or other technical terms such as 'roux', 'carders', 'trepanning', 'osmosis' and 'sphygmomanometer' – any words you would like to include, in fact.

Procedure

Each participant is given four pictures and a card from each section. They must make up a story linking the pictures and cards, and tell it to the group. They should be given a time limit, for example, five minutes, to invent the story.

Advice – it is often easier to establish the story ending first!

Speechmark

Spin doctor topic choice

Before embarking on this please have a look at Chapter 7 on lateral thinking for ideas to help your clients improve their underlying ability to think of topics for conversation. Here are some ideas that can follow, for actual topics for clients to try. You are aiming to get each participant to greet, to be greeted in response, and to add a comment, and also to be responded to.

Materials needed

- Eight small plain cards with the letter 'H' on them ('H' stands for 'How are you?').

- Smallish pictures that depict the types of topic very often heard in conversation:

  - eight small pictures of weather types (newspapers often have reasonable ones, or you can download them from the internet)

  - four pictures of families (magazines and colour supplements should yield good examples)

  - two pictures of footballers and two of other sportspeople

  - two pictures of people at work – Speechmark 'Occupations' cards are ideal, but if you don't have these you can usually get some good photos from magazines or newspapers

  - four short and preferably well-illustrated articles cut from local and national newspapers, which you or a client should read aloud so that everyone is aware of the drift of the piece. It is probably wise to avoid controversial front-page articles.

- An empty plastic bottle.

- A large table.

Completing the game

Place or stick the eight weather pictures in a large circle on the table, equally spaced.

Place the 'How are you?' cards between the weather pictures. These represent the topics of conversation most often referred to in most people's conversation.

Now add all of the other pictures, distributing them equally round the circle.

Procedure

Your clients sit round the table and take turns to have a mini-conversation.

Each turn consists of:

1 greeting someone else appropriately

2 being greeted in return

3 spinning the bottle, reading out the topic they have landed on and making a comment about that topic, addressing this to the same person as before

4 listening to the response.

For example, a group member says 'Hi' to another (and is responded to), then spins the bottle. If the bottle points towards 'Weather', the participant could say 'I've had enough of all this snow, but I must say it was nice to get out of college for a day and go tobogganing'. The person on the receiving end of the comment should respond accordingly.

Or, after the mutual greetings, suppose the pointer lands on an article about an oil spill. The comment could be: 'I wonder whether you have to be a qualified vet to clean the oil off the birds'.

Suppose the topic after the greeting is 'How are you?', then as well as asking that question, they could add: 'Is your arm better after that fall?' It's often worth making the point that in most conversation openers we do tend to ask 'How are you?', but usually this is just to get a positive 'I'm fine, thanks' type of answer; most people certainly do not want a long report on your health! If the 'How are you?' questions become too dominant in this game, just remove all but one of them.

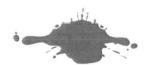

Give and take

A great role play game for learning negotiation techniques and how to make and accept compromises. There is a difference between negotiating and debating, in that negotiating does not produce one 'winner'; in fact a 'win–win' situation should be the outcome.

You need three clients for each role play, but it is preferable to have more than that in the group, to ensure that you can find people with opinions about each subject. People with Asperger's syndrome often find this activity very useful.

Materials needed

Storylines – you may need to invent some yourself, but most will come from local and national newspapers, and some from magazines. Keep the articles, especially if they have pictures. You are looking for stories that show a polarity of argument, and about which the clients already have opinions.

Getting started

Find out what the clients think about the stories. For example, in a story about shoplifting, probably one client will sympathise with the shoplifter and one will be more inclined to support the law. In an 'environmental issues' type of story, one client might favour banning private cars, while another might put personal freedom first. In an invented story, say about a sibling argument over which film to see at the cinema, a gangster-type movie or a cartoon, you will probably find a supporter for each side. Other invented scenarios might include 'Our college should have a uniform' or 'All junk food should be banned'.

The twist is that once you have established who favours which side of the argument, you ask them to argue the other person's case. This takes the heat out of the argument, making it into an exercise rather than just a quarrel. It also allows them to see the problem from the other person's point of view.

Procedure

As well as the proponents of each side of the argument, you need to have a judge. This figure asks each side in turn to do the following:

1 State their case, and then listen in silence to the statement from the other side.

2 Restate their case, adding anything else in the light of the other person's statement, and listen in silence to the other person's restatement.

3 Offer one compromise that the other side might accept, trying to be sure that both sides give some ground.

4 Agree on a course of action.

 Speechmark

The mediator now reiterates the problem, the compromises, and the conclusion reached.

It is wise to begin with distant, theoretical problems, and then gradually work towards problems which the clients might be familiar with.

Extra

If some of the clients are willing, once some hypothetical problems have been negotiated, it can be helpful to discuss any real issues that are communication based. For example, 'My houseparent often wants me to wash up when it's not my turn'. In this case the client actually involved in the disagreement should be an onlooker rather than a participant.

Charm dice

This is a useful and fun activity for a group, as an extension of work on conversation skills. It is a way to understand and practise the valuable skills of charm and politeness, and 'keeping one's cool' in awkward situations: either how to stay polite while fending off criticism or unkind remarks, or how to deal with compliments without getting flustered or appearing arrogant.

Quite often our clients are thought to be rude or thoughtless, when in fact the problem is that they just have not noticed other people's 'winning ways', or they have, but feel it is all too complicated for them to try to imitate.

Materials needed

- Two or more wooden, sponge or polystyrene cubes approximately 5cm across, obtainable from toyshops. Or, for the homemade version, make them from upholsterer's sponge as described in 'Question dice' earlier in this chapter.

- A narrow-tipped felt pen.

Completing the cubes

The 'rude cube' has potential conversation killers, atmosphere freezers or argument stimuli written on the sides. You will probably think of others, maybe more suitable to your particular clients, but here are some suggestions:

> *Oh no, not you again.*
>
> *Stop going on about it.*
>
> *You're late!*
>
> *What did you say that for?*
>
> *You are just copying me.*
>
> *I don't like you in that jacket.*

The other cube shows compliments; again, you would probably need to tailor them to your particular group:

> *You are so clever!*
>
> *Wow! You look fantastic!*
>
> *I like the way you talk.*
>
> *You have such good taste in clothes.*
>
> *I wish I could tell jokes as well as you can.*
>
> *Do tell me more, you are so interesting.*

Speechmark

Procedure

Take turns to roll the 'rude cube'. It's very important to be clear that the target is to emerge from the interaction in a charming and dignified way rather than descending into an argument or just storming off. It's also important, however, not to feel 'downtrodden' by trying to appease too much. The use of humour, or at least a smile, is invaluable in this situation. Here are some possible responses to the rude comments that the group might like to consider:

Oh no, not you again – 'Yes, sorry, you have to put up with me and my jokes again'.

Stop going on about it 'I'm sorry, I'm afraid it's one of my favourite topics. Let's talk about your favourite instead'.

You're late – 'I'm sorry, I thought we had decided on this time' or 'I'm sorry, I forgot the time'.

What did you say that for? – 'I didn't mean to upset you, I think we just misunderstood each other'.

You are just copying me – 'It's true that I would like to be as good as you at that. They say that imitation is the sincerest form of flattery'.

I don't like you in that jacket – 'Perhaps it doesn't really suit me that well, but I'm afraid I'm stuck with it as I can't afford another one at the moment'.

Now try rolling the 'compliments cube', and giving appropriate responses. Responding to compliments is often an even harder task than dealing with criticism or insults, because the client might find them embarrassing. The temptation is often to deny the compliment: 'Oh, I'm not really very good at it', or 'This is just an old dress, it's awful really'. These responses could make the person who gave the compliment feel quite insulted, as their kind opinion has been pushed aside. Often 'batting back' a compliment is the best bet, that is, returning flattery with a similar comment. Perhaps the following might be good responses, but again they are up for discussion:

You are so clever – 'Thank you, I do try to do my best. You've done really well too'.

Wow! You look fantastic – 'Thank you, it's so nice that you've noticed'.

I like the way you talk – 'Thank you, nice of you to notice and not mind my accent'.

You have such good taste in clothes – 'Thanks, what a cool thing to say'.

I wish I could tell jokes as well as you can – 'That is such a kind compliment'.

Do tell me more, you are so interesting – 'Thanks, it's nice of you to show interest'.

Extension activity

After discussing how to receive compliments, it might be a worthwhile opportunity to discuss giving them. The real key is to make the compliment specific, that is, rather than saying 'You look nice' it is often better received if you mention a particular aspect of the person's appearance, for example, 'I really like you in that top – the colour is just right on you'.

 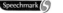

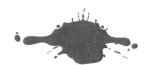

Similarly, it might be a good idea to discuss giving constructive criticism, for example, instead of 'You're late', it would be better to say 'I'm glad to see you, I was getting a bit worried that we'd made a mistake with the timing', or rather than 'I don't like you in that jacket' it might be better to say 'That jacket is OK, but I liked that other one even better'.

My news and yours

A great starter for every SLT session, this is a good way for clients to catch up on each other's news, and to rehearse the structure of a typical conversation outside of the clinical setting.

Materials needed

None, although you might like to jot down the clients' news for future reference.

Procedure

In turns, say what you have been doing since the last session. Encourage your clients to talk about their weekend, and add one other piece of news. Give them your news first, at least the first time you try this activity.

Now take it in turns to see if anyone can remember what was said.

Then the next client tells their news and again the others try to remember it, and so on around the circle.

As the clients progress, try this variation – all take turns to tell news, then after everyone has finished, consider each person in turn and everyone tries to remember their news. This is a harder task as the memorising will have been interrupted by others' news.

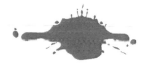

Other activities to help with conversation skills

Please see also:

1 For narrative skills: 'Life of Riley', 'Lucky dip reporting game' and 'So that's how that happened!' in Chapter 7 'Lateral thinking'.

2 For optimism: 'Every cloud', also in Chapter 7 'Lateral thinking'.

3 For phone conversations, try the 'Which service do you require?' activity in Chapter 4 'Listening skills'.

4 For topic choice, try 'News and weather round-up' in Chapter 8 'Memory'.

5 For general conversation technique, try 'Totem pole' in Chapter 15 'Wallcharts and decorations'.

6 For getting the right 'register' or social code, try the '"Formal and casual" board', also in Chapter 15 'Wallcharts and decorations'.

7 For informal commenting: 'Arty party' also in Chapter 15 'Wallcharts and decorations'.

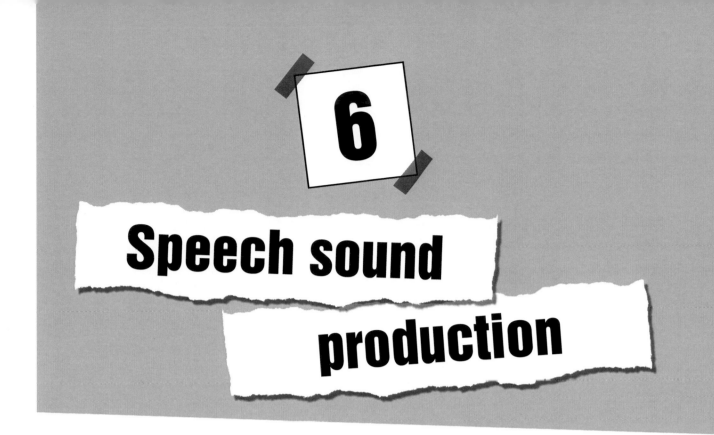

Speech sound production

Here's a reason to relish a trip to the dentist! Have you ever had extensive dental treatment involving, perhaps, root canal work? If you can bear to remember that for a moment, you may also remember the after effects of the local anaesthetic you were given (probably lignocaine or novocaine), which probably lasted no more than an hour or so. Temporarily you lacked sensitivity in part of your lip and/or tongue, and may have experienced a sensation of having a hugely swollen lip. You may have found it quite difficult to speak clearly.

Imagine a difficulty similar to yours, but with the speech difficulty lasting for much longer: how upsetting it would be to know that others are frequently misunderstanding what you say. Many of our clients would not experience such a profound, or any, sensation of numbness, but would still have a difficulty in sound production and with feedback or self-monitoring of their speech sounds.

It is likewise an eye opener to see members of staff at talks and workshops suddenly realising how difficult and frustrating communication must be for people with phonological difficulties. We demonstrate this difficulty without anaesthetic(!) by asking the staff to put three fingers in their mouths, that is, vertically, for maximum disruption to the speech apparatus, and then try to say something important (such as the name of a favourite pub!).

While some of our clients will struggle with their speech clarity so much that they might always need to augment speech with sign language or other forms of alternative and augmentative communication (AAC), many can be helped with articulation and phonology work. However, progress for some might take a long time, so it will be important to find lots of different ways to present what will essentially be the same thing.

There are already beautiful boxed games, photo cards and well-established exercises for speech and language therapists to use with clients who need to improve their speech production, but I venture to offer just a few more. They might add to your toolbox, address slightly different areas of speech work, or be used for the type of client who has outgrown some of the materials designed for younger people. They are also remarkably cheap!

Breathing gauges

This is a fun and simple way to encourage deeper breathing by clients of any age, as part of a course on breathing techniques — prerequisites for good speech. You can use it in one-to-one sessions or as a group activity. Take care not to encourage overly deep breathing, or your clients could become dizzy.

You could, of course, just use a tape measure, and make a note of the measurements at each of the exhaling and inhaling points, but this exercise makes a clearer visual message.

A word of warning regarding physical contact — don't do the measuring around the client's chest yourself, especially if the client is under 18. If they are unable to do their own measuring you should ask the parent/guardian or else abandon this idea.

Materials needed

- Narrow cotton tape.
- Felt tips of many colours, and biros.
- Wire coat hanger (if you are doing this activity with a group).

Making the strings

Cut a length of tape approximately 15cm longer than your client's approximate lower chest measurement.

Make a loop at one end – this is the bit that the client will hold while measuring themselves, and which will later become the attachment for hanging up on the coat hanger.

Forming the breathing gauges

The idea is to mark, in different colours, four points on the string that represent the client's chest measurement when they are fully exhaled, naturally inhaled, more deeply inhaled and fully inhaled.

Make sure the client understands the instructions about how to breathe out, and how deeply to breathe in – some practice may be needed, and you will need to demonstrate this activity as the client is doing it, to help them understand the procedure.

The tape needs to be pulled fairly tightly around the chest each time, preferably not over a coat or thick jumper.

Now ask the client to do the following, as demonstrated by you:

1   Breathe out fully, and mark this point on the tape, making a firm line across the tape to make it really clear.

2   Breathe in naturally, and add this new point to the tape.

3 Breathe in deeply, and again add this point.

4 Breathe in very deeply, and add this final point.

Take care over the possible issue of hyperventilation. Your client may need to have breaks between each breath.

Discuss the differences between the client's markings on their tape, and what this represents, and compare with your own results if appropriate.

You now have a baseline measurement for these four chest positions. If you are working as a group you will need to label the strings with the clients' names, because the idea is to keep them and remeasure later as a way to demonstrate improvement.

The coat hanger

Tie all the strings loosely on to the hanger so that you can remove them at the next or another session and see if there is any change. If or when there is an increase, just keep adding more colours.

If you have enough of these coloured strings, you can leave them on the hanger together, to make an interesting wall decoration. If you bind the coat hanger itself in brightly coloured wools you will have a decoration that is a real breath of fresh air!

Phonimals

Sometimes young clients working on articulation and phonology need a break from their usual speech sound work. This is a light-hearted way to relieve their work, but still keeping sound formation in mind.

Materials needed

- Small pillowcase or old fabric bag.

- Farm, pet and zoo animal toys. The bought varieties could be quite expensive, although I have found cheap ones at a warehouse store. Alternatively you can sometimes find suitable second-hand examples at car boot or jumble sales. Wash them well before use.

- Otherwise you can make the animals yourself, either before the session or with the client, and for this you will need:

  - lots of old gloves that you don't mind cutting up. It's the fingers you want, so cut them off. Fur-lined leather ones would be perfect, but even acrylic ones are OK

  - small card discs to stick on to the glove fingers

  - felt tip pens to decorate the discs with different animals' faces. The animals need to be the sorts that make noises that everyone would recognise, so: cat, dog, pig, cow, sheep, elephant, donkey, snake, owl, duck and bee, for example. Add some invented animals too, but decide together on the sound that animal makes. This will be a sound that fits in with your current phonology work (write the sound somewhere on the face to remind you which sound you chose).

Procedure

Place the 'animals' in the bag, and take turns to fumble inside it to find an animal and make the noise that animal makes, as clearly as you can. The other group members then join in with the same sound too (or just with you, if it's a one-to-one session). Try to be as accurate as you can with the animal sounds, and engineer things so that you can get some 'useful' articulation movements and sounds out of the game, as well as some that are just for fun.

Variation

The client picks out an animal without anyone else seeing it, and makes the sound for others to guess.

Phonbola

This is a fun addition to your phonological materials. You can use it as a one-to-one activity, or in a group.

Materials needed

- Big cylindrical glass jar – I've found that extra-large jars of pickled gherkins are quite easy to find for some reason – but you will need to find a keen gherkin eater to empty it for you! If your therapy room has an unforgiving floor you will need to find a plastic jar instead.

- Pen.

- Small pieces of thin, foldable card.

Making the game

Write words or phrases containing your client's target sound on the cards. Alternatively, if your client is a non-reader, draw little pictures, or you could use Widgit symbols.

Procedure

Simply place the folded cards in the jar, put the lid on, and roll it towards your client. They pick out a card and read it or name it, trying to be as clear as possible.

Variation

The client picks out a card and then makes a sentence containing the 'jar word'.

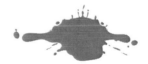

Click click

I used to play a game like this when I was a child, at Brownies! The original game aimed to help all members of the Brownie pack to learn each other's names (and of course you could still use it in that way if you are working with a group needing practice at remembering names).

This variation seeks to help with syllable division. Once a client has learned to divide words into syllables it becomes much easier to elicit medial sounds. Also it can sometimes be helpful to work with syllable division with dysfluent clients, if you are trying to even out their speech rhythms.

Materials needed

Pictures, symbols or written labels of the items to be named.

Procedure

Each member of the group is given a two-syllable word, and a picture of the item which they leave on the table so that everyone can be reminded of one another's words (unless you also want to work on memory). They need to practise saying their own and each other's words clearly, with two distinct beats, before you start the game.

Words such as 'apple', 'pencil', 'robin', 'gravy', 'England', 'donkey', 'speakers', 'mobile', 'iPod' and 'wallet' would all be fine. Nouns are best, as they are easier to illustrate.

Establish a beat. To get started this would be two clicks of the fingers, two claps, and then two non-words with two syllables, for example, 'dah-dah, dee-dee'. So, click – click – clap – clap – dah-dah, dee-dee. Repeat this several times – slowly – until the idea of the rhythm seems to be established.

Now explain that where the dah-dah, dee-dee sounds were used you are going to put the words they have learned, and that they will take it in turns to click twice, clap twice, say their own word, and then any other person's, all in rhythm. So: click – click – clap – clap – apple – pencil. The 'pencil' person repeats the procedure: click – click – clap – clap – pencil – mobile. Then the 'mobile' person takes over. Continue until everyone has had a turn.

Sometimes people get flustered when they have to think who to pass the turn to, so to avoid their embarrassment you could remove the element of choice, by just passing the turns to the left until they become more used to the game.

Once they become rhythmical with two-syllable words you can progress to three-syllable words. These will be preceded by three clicks and three claps. To start with, it's best to choose words that have the stress on the first syllable, for example, 'elephant', 'Portugal', 'animal', 'broccoli', 'parachute', 'caramel', 'cucumber'. So the three clicks and claps will be accentuated in that way also, that is, CLICK – click – click – CLAP – clap – clap – parachute – caramel.

Speechmark

If you want to use three-syllable words with the stress on the second syllable, try to group them together for a separate round, so that the rhythm works well. These might include 'computer', 'Ferrari', 'tombola', 'piranha', 'tomato', 'potato'. You'll also need to adjust the accentuation with the clicking and clapping.

As the group becomes comfortable with the game you can try four- or even five-syllable words with the appropriate click and clap formation.

Extended version

You can extend this even further by trying phrases or short sentences of equal syllable length and with comparable accentuation: 'on the phone', 'just in time', 'by the way', 'time for tea' or 'give me strength' for example.

Limericks

This is a speech activity either for a group of fairly able, older clients to write themselves (or co-write), or for children and other less confident people to have written for them. The use of limericks helps to develop rhythm, and appreciation of rhyme. When spoken aloud these poems need to be articulated very clearly, so they help with speech difficulties. They can also be a good-humoured way to bring communication problems out in the open so that they can be tackled. You will need to be able to write limericks fairly easily yourself, in order to help the clients, but here are some tips to help you.

What is a limerick?

Limericks follow this basic pattern and beat:

A tiddly tiddly pom

A tiddly tiddly pom

A tiddly dee

A tiddly dee

A tiddly tiddly pom.

There is often an extra beat or even two extras on the first, second and last lines.

The first, second and fifth lines need to rhyme, and the third and fourth lines also need a separate rhyme. You will find excellent examples of limericks in books of humorous poetry, especially by Edward Lear.

How do you write a limerick?

You'll often find it's easier to complete the limerick if you start with the last word – the one which is usually the most important, as then you can manipulate the first two lines to arrive at the best rhyme. Here are some examples of limericks that I've co-written with clients.

This one was used as a way of affirming Sue's opinions, thereby promoting confidence in expressing herself:

There was a young lady called Sue

Who came down by taxi from Kew.

She hated school curry

From pizza she'd hurry

But chose all the time to eat stew.

This one was therapy-orientated, but with Ed's agreement:

There once was a student called Ed

It was hard to hear what he said.

He spoke oh so quickly

 Speechmark

Your ears got quite tickly

But now he speaks slowly instead.

Here are a couple you might be able to use as frameworks for your clients if you tweak the names. Make sure that they are happy to do this. If you have built a good relationship with your clients you'll be able to use humour in this way to help them.

Miranda had trouble with s

So she struggled to say her address.

But she's learnt some new speech

For the farm, town or beach

And we smile, because she'll impress.

Or maybe …

Our Benji did not like to look

In the eyes of a friend, staff, or cook,

Now he's trying to peer

Not at eyes, but quite near,

And he no longer hides in his book.

You can, of course, write other styles of poetry or rap for or with your clients.

Speechmark

Other activities to help with speech sound production

Please see also:

1 The 'Variation' section of 'Speedy categories' in Chapter 9 'Vocabulary'.

2 'Sound effects' in Chapter 4 'Listening skills'.

3 'Which service do you require?' in Chapter 4 'Listening skills'.

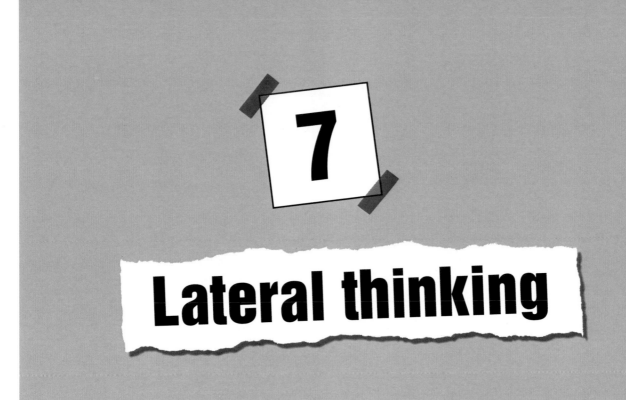

Lateral thinking

'Whatever shall I say next?' must be a thought that has occurred to most of us at times in conversations with unforthcoming people at social occasions. Sometimes a silence can be friendly and comfortable, especially with someone we know well, and in this case no 'filler' is needed. However, not all conversational silences are easy; sometimes they are awkward or uncomfortable, and you can feel desperate to think of some topic that will keep things going. For the person with limited lateral thinking the task is even harder.

This chapter does not set out to make a list of conversation topics – see Chapter 5 'Conversation skills' for further help with that   but instead it gives ideas for working on the client's underlying ability to think laterally.

If you have never tried it, you might begin this work with your clients by asking them to think of as many ideas as they can for using, say, an empty drink can. At first, especially if their diagnosis is somewhere on the autism spectrum, they may come up with only one or two uses. But now ask them to pretend to be an artist, a musician or a hunter and do the same task. They will almost always, as I have found, arrive at several more ideas.

So we can see that it is possible to help people with this problem, and on the following pages are some further ideas to extend this work. The exercises should also prove to be good fun, and can be used to lighten the mood of a session.

Life of Riley

This is a lateral thinking activity for a group of fairly able children or young teenagers. It also helps to develop narrative skills. The idea is to explain how the cars could have got into such a state. Extra praise should be given for the funniest or most outlandish ideas.

Materials needed

As many battered old toy cars as you can find, the worse their condition the better.

Alternatively, and more appropriate for older clients, would be pictures of real 'old bangers'. You can get these from a specialist magazine on stock car racing. You could, of course, use other old vehicles such as buses, trains and motorbikes.

Procedure

Hand a car, or picture of one, to each client, who then inspects the car and thinks up a story to explain the current condition of the vehicle, and tells this to the whole group.

You can get the ball rolling yourself, for example, describing how a vehicle started life as a family car, and was stolen and used as a getaway car, or got left in a beach car park when the tide came in. It was later sold to a new driver as a first car, but kept being badly parked, bumping into posts. It might even have been taken to a safari park and 're-engineered' by a monkey.

Finally, you can decide and describe the fate of the car: perhaps the plan will be to start a new life, after being repaired and repainted, or to be crushed and made into saucepans! Try to end the car's 'life' on a reasonably positive note.

'Also for ...'

This is a lateral thinking game for a group of clients of any age.

Materials needed

The objects required for this activity are usually readily to hand in any office, or you can supplement them with common kitchen utensils, handbag contents or other items.

Procedure

Pick up an item, for example, a pencil or a paperclip, and think of an alternative use for it. Each client just thinks of one new use, then passes it on to the next person who does the same. When no one can think of any more uses, pick up a new item.

The new uses can be as wild and wacky as you like, for instance, a pencil could be used as a plant support, a chopstick, a hair decoration, a window prop, or a stick for a paper windmill. A paperclip could be used as a hairgrip, an earring, a link from a paperclip necklace, a tool for extracting something stuck in a crevice, or something to stick on the back of a photo (ie to be picked up by a magnet).

You can take the opportunity during this game to make the point that 'two heads are better than one', that is, that if we all pool our ideas we can have better results (and this links into friendship skills).

Seasonal variation

Think of alternative uses for Christmas items, for example, tinsel, decorated cake board, Father Christmas hat, stocking, pudding basin and mince pie case.

So that's how that happened!

This is a lateral thinking activity for a group of fairly able clients. It is based on the idea of explaining how something improbable could have come about, and is great fun and very funny sometimes. We were playing this game once when the Ofsted inspector arrived. He was persuaded to join in and entertained us amusingly for a good five minutes!

Materials needed

List of unlikely circumstances, such as the examples listed below, written on small pieces of paper, folded, and put in a hat.

Procedure

Clients are asked to make up a story, the end point of which is the unlikely circumstance written on their piece of paper. They are allowed a few minutes to think of their story, perhaps while tea break is going on.

Suggestions for unlikely circumstances

… so that is how I came to arrive at my interview for the office job wearing muddy boots.

… so that is how our college came to be used as an animal shelter for the weekend.

… so that is how I realised I had dyed my friend's hair purple.

… so that is how I found myself under the table at a stranger's wedding reception wearing my swimming costume.

… so that is how the inspector came to be sitting on a plate of ice cream.

… so that is how I found myself on a rocket to the moon.

… so that is how I found myself having to spend the night in an empty multi-storey car park.

… so that is how it was my fault that the Prime Minister came to rip his trousers.

… so that is how I came to be shopping in my pyjamas and a tall hat.

… and so that's how that happened!

Lucky dip reporting game

This game helps to develop lateral thinking and narrative skills in fairly able clients. The idea is for the clients to become 'reporters' who provide a main idea, and then give a few details to go with a newspaper headline that they have picked out of a container. Playing this game also provides an opportunity for you to suggest that keeping up to date with, and being able to talk about, real news can be a good conversation skill.

Materials needed

- Plenty of headlines cut out of newspapers. Vague themes are best, rather than headlines that restrict the reporter to one particular story.

- Some sort of container – a basket, hat or bag, for example.

- Small envelopes.

Preparing the game

Place each the headline in an envelope. This is preferable to just putting them straight into the container, because otherwise you risk them getting ripped. Also, in this way the headline can be kept private to the 'reporter', avoiding others chipping in.

Procedure

Clients are asked to pick out an envelope, look at the headline, and then provide a short report to follow it. Request that they keep the headline to themselves until they have a rough idea of their report.

Suggest that they then read out their headline, and follow it with a main theme, and then just two or three details.

It's good if you as therapist go first. Let's say the headline reads:

Phew! What a scorcher!

You could give a main theme:

Temperatures reached 35 degrees centigrade in Gloucestershire today

and then supply three details:

Farmer John Smith had to keep his cattle indoors today to stop them getting heatstroke. He put the hoses on to spray them. He blamed global warming for this problem.

Praise clients for reports of the right length. Those who tend to 'ramble' will benefit from having to be short and to the point, while those who tend to offer only one word as a response will have to elaborate.

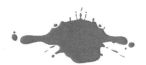

Shadows

This is a lateral thinking game that involves drawing as well as describing. It is suitable for a group, or could be used for a one-to-one session. You must have access to a photocopier if you want to do this activity.

Materials needed

- Paper.

- Pens and pencils.

- Access to a photocopier.

- Odd objects that are flat enough to go in a photocopier. These could be:

  - several paperclips grouped together

  - some pressed flowers or leaves

  - a pair of scissors

  - scrunched-up piece of net

  - a squiggle of string

  - a few buttons or sequins

  - bits of torn paper.

Preparation

Place the odd objects on the platen of the photocopier, but off centre so that the resulting image has room for further additions to be drawn on. Make enough copies of the odd objects for everyone in the group to have one of each.

Procedure

Try to arrange it so that the participants cannot see each other's work.

Ask them to finish the pictures by drawing an addition to the image on the paper. For example, the flat image of a pair of scissors can be transformed into the jaws of a crocodile if it faces one way, or into a face if the fingerholds are made to represent the eyes. The clients should add a title to the finished result.

Now they describe their work of art to the group.

Speechmark

Alternative odd one out

This is a lateral thinking game for a group of fairly able clients who must already have grasped the notion of the traditional 'odd one out'. This alternative idea is that the clients stretch their minds to seek the less obvious 'oddities'. This can help with observational skills. The core ability to think laterally is also, I believe, helpful in being able to think of conversational topics. I have also found that a good discussion about difference, similarity or uniqueness can emerge from this.

Materials needed

'Odd one out' cards or sets of objects that show easy and obvious odd ones out – you could use themed objects such as cutlery, plastic farm animals, tools and make-up.

Procedure

Place a number of objects in a theme together: say four red toy cars and one of a different colour, and add a red lipstick or a red flower. It is a moot point whether the differently coloured car or the flower is the odd one out. Discuss the answers as a group or each person does one example.

You could try office equipment, all but one item beginning with the letter *s* (scissors, Sellotape, pencil, stapler and stamp) and one other thing beginning with *s* (eg scarf). The pencil is odd because it doesn't begin with s, and the scarf is also odd in not being office equipment.

What about party and party games equipment – balloons, straws, whistles, party blowouts and crisps, and a recorder. Is the recorder odd (non-party) or are the crisps odd (edible)?

And so it goes on.

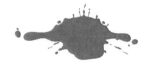

Every cloud

This activity has two main purposes: lateral thinking practice, and how to be optimistic. Clients who are working on idiom will also learn the meaning of the expression 'Every cloud has a silver lining'.

Materials needed

- List of problems.
- Paper and pens.

Procedure

Write a problem at the top of the page, for example, 'Amy broke her ankle but ...' Now, as a group, brainstorm some positive points about such a situation. These could be: she found that her true friends rallied round to help her; she found out different ways of doing things (like bouncing down the stairs on her bottom, and drinking her tea beside the kettle rather than carrying it to her table); she learned to use crutches, and in so doing her arms got stronger; people wrote funny things on her plaster; she was given lots of flowers; and she had time to learn to knit.

Other hypothetical problems and positive points might include:

There was a power cut (but – we ate by candlelight; we had a log fire; we teamed up with others and had a bonfire; we saved a bit on electricity).

We missed the train (but – while waiting we took the opportunity to have a coffee in the station café; we caught a later one which was a through train; we spent another day on holiday).

Our car broke down (but – at last we were able to benefit from all those years of paying in to the RAC; two of us could go and get everyone an ice cream; it made us decide to buy a new car; it made us decide to sell the car and use public transport instead).

Faith failed her driving test (but – she was able to have a bit more practice before driving alone so was a safer driver in the end; she didn't need her own car yet, so could save on petrol money; one less driver means a bit less pollution; she shared a lift with someone who became a friend).

When you have tackled some hypothetical situations you might feel that the group can look at some actual problems of their own. It's best to stick to fairly light problems that will pass in time rather than examining deeper difficulties.

Variation

A variation on this game is an old party game called 'The good news and the bad news'. In this version one person states a piece of good news, for example, 'The good news is that it's a sunny day'. The next person begins their statement with 'But the bad news is that ...', and adds a point such as 'we might get sunburn'. The next person adds 'But the good news is that ...', and might suggest 'I have some excellent sun cream and a long-sleeved tee-shirt', and so on round the circle.

 Speechmark

What on earth...?

A handy addition to your materials for developing lateral thinking skills. The game is suitable for a group of four or five. It links to the 'Also for …?' game, but is subtly different in that rather than describe other uses for an object whose purpose you already know, this time you are casting about, trying to think of what the original purpose could have been.

Materials needed

- Strong (preferably fabric) bag – size depends on your choice of contents.

- Funny objects. This is the main challenge in preparing for the game, in that ideally you would provide objects which no one else will have seen before. You may find, as I did, that there are all sorts of peculiar items (often Auntie's Christmas presents!) in your kitchen drawer, for example, honey scoops, ice lolly moulds or parts of coffee makers. A tool chest may also yield some weird things, and parts of packaging. My lovely friend and assistant Julia, a part-time upholsterer who also used to own a flock of sheep, provided some items whose original uses I found impossible to guess – perhaps wisely! Even broken items (but not sharp or otherwise hazardous) will be fine.

Procedure

In turns, each group member picks one item from the bag. Spend some time examining the item, and then describe one or more uses for it. Miming, to clarify the meaning, is to be encouraged.

This game is good fun, and is comfortable for everyone, as the answers are hidden in obscurity, so no one would be expected to know. Often it can be hilarious too.

Incredible powers

This activity is very popular with children, but fun for younger teenagers too. It has a link with the many films about superheroes who have special powers. You are trying to elicit imaginative ideas in general and particularly about clients' positive and altruistic aims, so, if possible, steer them gently away from anything too much related to weaponry or world destruction!

Materials needed

None, although you might want to encourage the clients to draw themselves with their incredible power, in which case paper and felt tips would be needed.

Procedure

Ask the clients to think of an incredible power or talent they wished they had and how they would use it. They might need several minutes to think of something, but then in turn they describe it, mime it, or draw it for the group to discuss.

If they are stumped for ideas, here is a list that they might choose from, or use for inspiration for other, better ones. In this case you would just prompt them with: 'If you had one of these talents which would it be, and why?'

The ability to:

- become invisible
- be someone else for a day
- travel at the speed of sound
- see through walls
- fly or float in the air
- climb up vertical walls
- see in the dark
- use supersonic hearing
- breathe fire
- swim underwater without the need to breathe
- lift tremendous weights
- change shape
- turn anything to ice by pointing at it
- stop time
- resist bullets and knives with your armoured skin
- make crying babies giggle
- heal broken limbs with a touch of your finger
- repair machinery by whistling at it
- change the weather
- talk to animals
- bounce
- communicate telepathically
- wiggle your nose to do housework
- stick anything to anything else
- turn silver into gold
- see into the future.

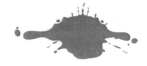

Other ideas to help with lateral thinking skills

Please see also:

1   For sophisticated lateral thinking skills, 'Question dice' in Chapter 5 'Conversation skills'.

2   For more high-powered lateral thinking, once your clients are working on conversational idea-generation, try 'Just a minute', also in Chapter 5 'Conversation skills'.

Speechmark

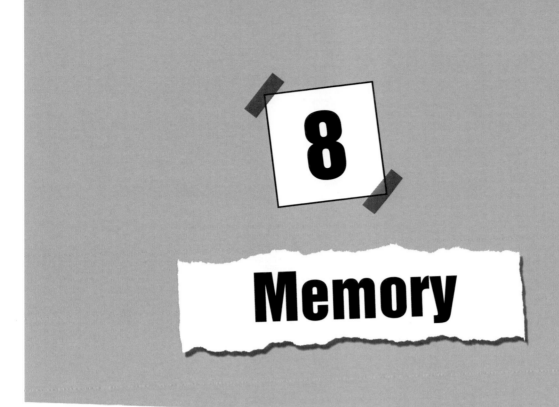

8

Memory

There are many great theorists on memory who have written copiously on the subject, and it is not my brief to go down the theory track in any great detail. Well-established activities for promoting memory skills include the following:

1 For auditory memory:

People with a lowered working or auditory memory may have enormous problems in retaining what has just been said to them, some even struggling to remember the first part of a sentence by the time the end of it is reached.

Active listening is a key skill for the client to use. This means focusing exclusively on the speaker, silently repeating the words, and using mental pictures if that helps. Above all, it is important that the client feels able to ask for repetition or clarification.

Also it is important to make sure that those working with such clients are aware of the difficulty, so that they can use the technique of 'chunking and checking', that is, breaking long sentences into short 'chunks', and then observing or asking, to 'check' that the client has really understood and retained whatever was said.

2 For short-term memory:

The short-term memory lasts a little longer. Here 'short-term' applies to both visual and auditory memory types. Useful activities include the following:

Games such as the old favourite 'Kim's game', where items are placed on a tray and looked at for some moments, then one item is secretly removed and the client(s) must remember what used to be there.

'Pelmanism' is the game where pairs of cards are placed face down on the table, and muddled up, then picked up two at a time and kept if they match, play then passing to the next player.

Then there are the cumulative 'circle' games, such as 'In my suitcase I packed … (add an item such as sunglasses)', which the next participant repeats and adds to, thus: 'In my case I packed sunglasses and pyjamas'. Now the next repeats and adds, in the same way, and so on until it becomes too difficult to remember. Other cumulative games will be visual rather than auditory, and include those such as the excellent 'Addabout' which I found in Dr Wendy Rinaldi's *Social Use of Language Programme*, and used as part of that course. (In that game one person performs an action, such as waving, which the next participant copies and adds to – wave, jump; then the next might add a shoulder shrug after repeating the wave and the jump, and so on.)

Story CDs with subsequent questions are helpful but expensive – you can find stories with questions, which you could read out to your clients. English textbooks for schools are good sources for useful stories.

3 For long-term memory:

Long-term memory is our store of useful information, such as people's names, or what happened when. Visual memory is important here too: for a client who finds it difficult to put names to faces it's equally important to remember the face as well as the name.

Keeping a journal or diary can help to fix a memory, as can making a labelled photograph album. Some clients like to learn something by heart, for example, a joke or poem (especially good if they have made it up themselves).

Writing down some key words connected with a film, book or play will help in storing the plot and characters.

Some of the following memory games are variations on old games, and some are inventions that I use frequently.

Car logo Pelmanism

A variation of the traditional memory game, particularly useful for clients who are keen on cars. It is suitable for a group, or could be used for a one-to-one session.

Materials needed

- As many pictures of cars and their logos as you can get your hands on. Two of each are needed. (Weekend newspaper colour supplements or other car magazines are good sources.)

- Card. Index cards, or half-size index cards. 'Taskmaster' blank cards would give a superior effect.

Preparation

Learn or make a note of the car manufacturer corresponding to each logo, or write on the cards. Stick one logo or one car image on each card. Note: you can vary the level of difficulty in picture pairing, choosing to show either identical images – two cars or two logos – or perhaps the logo on one card and an image of the car itself on the other.

Procedure

Place the cards face up on the table. The number presented at a time is up to you, but I have found it best to start with three pairs to convey the idea, and then build up. (For some clients you may end up with as many as 15 pairs on the table.) Turn the cards over and muddle them up.

Turn two cards over. If they are a pair (ie two cars, or two logos, or logo with matching car), the player keeps them. If not, turn them back over again.

Play passes to the next person. The winner is the one with the most pairs.

Alternative game – a version of 'Kim's game'

Place just one of each of the card pairs (ie so that all the cards are different) face up on the table. The number presented at a time is up to you. I have found it best to start with three cards to convey the idea, and then build up.

Turn the cards over and muddle them up. Take away one card, hide it, and turn the others face up again. The client must decide which one has gone.

You could of course, take away more than one card at a time.

You can also use these cards to play Snap.

Variation

Instead of car logos, you could use clothing logos (Nike, Adidas) or small pictures of cosmetic items (nail varnish, shampoo) – or the ever-popular chocolate bars! In fact you can use anything that fits on your cards and is of interest to your clients.

Incidentally, some of the supermarkets produce good photos of food and other items in their leaflet handouts and recipe cards, so this can provide another source of (free) pictures.

True story

This memory activity helps clients to listen, and to learn something about each other. The true story could be something about their biography, or maybe an event that took place last weekend, for example, a barbecue, or a trip to a zoo. It also requires the person telling their story to plan something reasonably coherent, for which they may need some help. If your clients prefer, they can tell made-up stories. It is best for a group of four teenagers or adults.

Materials needed

None.

Procedure

Person A tells their story, which should last approximately half a minute. Person B repeats the story as exactly as possible, trying to use the same words and inflections. Person C mimes it. Person D tells it again, but as a character might, for example, an old woman or a reporter. Together try to think of some questions that would extend the information originally given.

Now person B tells their story, and the procedure is repeated.

When everyone has told their story, try to remember Person A's story.

The outcome should demonstrate that if the clients really focus on other people's news or biographies, they can remember them, and use them to form part of a conversation. The point can also be made that if the story is remembered, it can be referred to at a later date, showing interest, and possibily helping to build a friendship.

Speechmark

Remembering in threes

This is a memory game to pounce on if your client can sort items into categories. It is best for a one-to-one therapy session. It is a huge morale booster for clients who feel that they have difficulties in the area of memory.

Materials needed

- Pictures of nouns. You need nouns in categories, for example, vegetables, drinks, clothes, tools, flowers and furniture. You could also try more general categories, such as things you can buy at a chemist's shop, at a newsagent's or in a shoe shop (name the shops on your high street). If you are looking for free pictures, I recommend the general categories as you will be able to cut pictures out of catalogues or promotional material.

- Cards – 'Taskmaster' blanks, index cards, or pieces of card that you have cut to approximately postcard size.

- Glue.

Preparation

Stick the pictures on the cards. Make sure you have at least three pictures in each category, and at least three categories. In fact, five or six in a category and nine categories would make it a much better activity as you will then be able to repeat the exercise several times without using the same pictures.

Procedure

You are aiming to help your client remember nine items. This seems a lot, but there is a trick to this type of memory.

Show your client nine cards, three pictures in three categories. Let's say category A is a banana, an apple and an orange; category B is a hammer, a saw and a screwdriver; category C is a box of plasters, a bottle of vitamin tablets and a tube of toothpaste. Present the cards in a muddled heap and ask the client to sort them into fruits, tools and things you get at a chemist's. Have each grouping of cards placed apart from the next group so that they are distinct.

Spend time discussing the three cards in each category, for example, whether they like the fruits; whether they have ever used any of the tools (also mime the actions, eg hammering); why they might need plasters, vitamins and toothpaste.

Now proceed as for Kim's game, that is, turn the cards over, muddle them up, and remove one card without letting the client see what it is. Turn the other cards back over and ask the client to sort them again into the three groups. In this way you are helping them to narrow down the possibilities: the chances for remembering the missing card are much higher.

Praise is given, the missing card is replaced and the whole process is repeated, but this time removing a different card. You might need to repeat several times with the same set of

 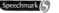

cards, but then, or at the next session, try a different set. Aim towards memorising the types of items on a shopping list, so finer categories will be needed – things on the meat counter, on the bakery shelf, in the freezer, and so on.

The outcome should demonstrate that if the client organises the things they have to remember, they can hold a lot more in their heads.

One warning: some clients will not be able to remember even three items. An easier version will use actual objects that can be held, and only present two items (exactly as for an easy Kim's game). Gradually build up to three items and then work towards two sets of two, and then two sets of three, items.

Menu game

In a café I sometimes visit with my family, there is a waiter who remembers everyone's orders without writing them down. When he returns with the various meals, he unfailingly places each dish in front of the right person. When I asked him how he was able to do this he said that he forms a mental picture of each person eating their chosen meal. In the clinical situation we have tried a similar approach to memory exercises, with good results.

The game is all the more motivating because the menu is devised by the group themselves – calling on their abilities to think laterally and work cooperatively. It is also a useful activity for those working on independence or life skills. In addition, the role play element can be fun. It is suitable for a group of about three or four clients.

Materials needed

- Menu forms – you can photocopy the one on page 103, or make your own.
- Pens.
- Biscuits (at your discretion).

Devising the menu

Each group member thinks of two or three dishes for each course and jots them down on scrap papers that are then pooled. (It's a good idea to do this part anonymously.) On examination of the types of food chosen, the group decide together whether the hypothetical eating place is an upmarket restaurant or inclines more towards the 'greasy spoon' end of the market, and whether you are going to offer two or three courses. If you choose to have starters the game is much more difficult because the waiter may have to remember two courses for each person. Once you have arrived at a reasonable range of dishes you can write the list down on some of the forms. At this point you may like to stop, leaving the ordering part for the next session.

Procedure

Begin by explaining that although real waiting staff usually write the orders down, you are going to try to remember the orders without such an aid. Then tell the group that memorising the list of orders will be much easier if they associate a face with a meal. Take turns to be the waiter and hand out the completed menus. The other players each request their starter and the waiter repeats each person's order immediately, and then repeats the whole group order. If the waiter feels able, they then repeat the process with the main course and, if really confident, will repeat the whole group's starter and main course. Now the waiter goes out of the room, and then returns with as many plates as they can mime carrying! They then mime placing each dish in front of the correct customer, stating what the dish actually is. They wait for a moment before miming clearing the table, exiting the room again, and coming back with the main courses, stating what they are as they place them, as before.

Serving the dessert will be the last part of their task, and is carried out in the same way.

You might decide to have different waiters for each course if the activity seems to be too difficult, or if others are keen to have their go.

You might want to offer biscuits to the group after all that talk of food!

Variations

This is well received by 18-year-olds and above – instead of a café with its food menu and waiter, you can conjure up a pub, with a list of possible drinks and a person buying a round. Each member requests a drink, and the person buying must remember which consumer requested which drink. Add peanuts and different flavours of crisps and you will have an excellent – and useful – memory game.

Younger children could have a beach café with ice creams and soft drinks.

The Hippo and Campus
Menu

Snacks

Sandwiches – egg and cress; tuna mayo; ham; cheese and pickle – £ 2.00

Sausage rolls – or vegetarian sausage roll – £1.50

Soups all at £2.50, served with a roll

Tomato

Pea and ham

Chicken noodle

Main Courses all at £3.50 served with salad

Spaghetti Bolognaise

Sausage and chips

Fish and chips

Vegetarian quiche

Pizza

Desserts all at £2.00

Ice cream (several flavours available, just ask)

Chocolate gâteau

Crème brûlée

Fruit salad

Apple pie

Cheese and biscuits

Beverages

Coffees – £1.50

Teas – £1.00

Herbal teas – £1.25

Soft drinks – Coke, Lemonade, J2O, Appletiser – prices on request

Other drinks to order from the bar

News and weather round-up

This is a useful memory exercise as well as a helpful way of demonstrating how topical events can enrich conversation. It is not an easy task; most people listen to the weather forecast and promptly forget most of what was said. As far as the news is concerned they are more successful, but not brilliant. (Try testing it on yourself — be honest, it wasn't easy, was it?) This exercise really needs forward planning as you should have some 'old news' to practise with at first.

Materials needed

- Two recordings of the news and weather, one from some time ago (preferably a month or more back) and one very recent one. It's best to use news that is not too upsetting or disturbing.

- Whatever recording and playback devices you have: maybe an MP3 player or mobile phone. Or for better quality, record sound clips off the internet and download electronically to an MP3 player.

Procedure

Play the 'old news' first. Ask for a volunteer to repeat the main headline.

Now ask other group members for any further points they remember. Play the news back again and see how much was remembered.

Now try the weather forecast. See if anyone can remember the forecast for the local area and then see if the weather for other areas can be recalled.

Repeat the whole exercise using a recent broadcast.

The trick, of course, is careful and active listening.

Extra

Make the point that knowing what is in the news will be a valuable asset for making contributions in conversations, especially if your client has the problem of not being able to think of topics to talk about.

Have a short discussion about the main or most interesting points of the news, and see if anyone has any opinions they would be willing to share.

Name game

This is a help for clients who find it hard to remember people's names, or lack confidence in using them. For fuller therapeutic value, it is important to introduce this game and draw it to a close carefully so that clients don't go away feeling that they have difficulty with this task. I always point out to the clients at the start that most people have some degree of difficulty in remembering names. This game can be done as a group or as an individual exercise.

Materials needed

- Blank cards – index cards or postcards are good as they are big enough to hold a decent-sized picture, or you can cut your own from any card.

- Cut-out magazine or newspaper pictures, of people of varying ages and types. Outlandish characters are memorable, and so are those performing an activity. Have about 30 pictures available for the clients to choose from, although you will probably use only five at a time.

- Glue.

- Pen.

- Lined paper.

Making the game

Stick the pictures on the cards. This can be done within the group session as a cooperative exercise, taking turns with the scissors and glue, and using the opportunity for a social chat as you work.

Write a number in a corner of each picture card and a corresponding number down the side of the lined paper. The numbered lined paper will be your record of the names chosen in the next stage of the game.

Choosing the names

With your clients, choose names that you feel suit the people in the photos, for example, for a man photographed with a prize fish you might like the name Mr Pike; a pretty young girl might be Jenny Sweet; an older lady seen at a craft market might be Mrs Woolly; and a boy photographed in the rain might be Ron Mac. Make a note on your numbered paper of the corresponding names. Go over the names and photos several times with the clients. Don't try to tackle more than a few names at a time – overloading may end in too much of a struggle. The idea is that they will learn the skill of selecting a detail from a person's appearance or lifestyle which reminds them of the person's name.

Procedure

A few minutes after making the name choices, present the picture cards one at a time, and ask the clients – either all together as a group or individually – to attempt to recall the names. To make the task harder, the recall attempt can take place after another activity, and again at the following session, and again several weeks later. As time goes on and the clients learn the names, you can introduce more and more new photos and corresponding names.

We found that the clients were pleasantly surprised at how easy it became to remember names when they were associated with the characters' idiosyncrasies or occupations.

It's a good idea to make a note of which set of clients have invented these names (use the lined sheet with the list of names chosen). You will need a new sheet of lined paper each time you play the game with a new set of clients. Alternatively, you could decide on a list of names which you will keep permanently.

Taking the name-learning further

The next step is to think of actual people who the clients are in some way connected with. Ideally you will have photos of these people, and can then discuss which aspects of their appearance, job or hobbies you can use as memory stimuli.

You can mention four extra name recall tips:

1 The client should repeat the name aloud when the person has just been introduced.

2 The client should consider phonological aspects of the name, for example, rhyme: the name Freja rhymes with layer. There is also alliteration as with Ozzy Osbourne.

3 The client should say the name several times silently to themselves, and use it a lot in conversation when they have just been introduced.

4 They should later write down the name and the memorable feature of the person, and keep this document. This will be a great confidence booster ready for the next time that they meet that person.

Other activities to help with memory skills

Please see also:

1 'Click click', in Chapter 6 'Speech sound production'.

2 'My news and yours', in Chapter 5 'Conversation skills'.

3 'Speedy categories', in Chapter 9 'Vocabulary'.

107

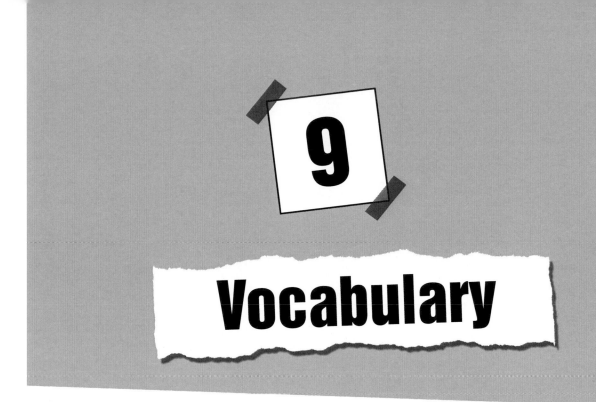

9

Vocabulary

If you have ever visited another country and struggled to remember the vocabulary you thought you had learned at school, you'll begin to understand how frustrating it would be not to be able to think of the words you need when you are speaking in your own language. In the same way, you might sometimes forget the name of a capital city, a type of rock formation, or a film star whose name you need for a quiz. That 'tip of the tongue' experience could be a frequent annoyance for clients who have trouble in storing and retrieving a word from their vocabulary.

Do you remember a comedy sketch on TV in which the setting was a library, where the books were classified by colour rather than in the more conventional categories? There may have been a certain logic in that method if you happened to know the colour of the book you were seeking! However, it does seem to save time if the books are arranged more logically, by fiction or non-fiction, by type and then by author, and finally by first letter of the title. There are also systems in the library to link the categories, so that an author who writes both fiction and non-fiction can be easily found in both.

It seems that most of us store words in our inner lexicons in a similarly logical way; in several types of categories including semantic and phonological forms. These help us to home in on the target word. We can also make 'cross-references' in our brains, as they do in a library, to make the whole process more accurate. They say that the English language has the largest vocabulary of any in the world, so storing and cross-referencing words has to be carried out extra carefully. It's important to store words in more than one category because otherwise you can get very odd alternatives chosen, for example, 'It's something woolly so it must be a sheep', when in fact the word you were seeking was 'cardigan'. It's a bit like that philosophical point about proving that a dog is a cat – 'A dog is an animal with four legs, a cat is an animal with four legs, so a dog must be a cat'!

There is already information about the way in which vocabulary development takes place, but my brief is not to go down the theoretical route myself. Instead, my advice would be to look at the excellent books by Sadie Lewis in this area on both theory and practice.

In this chapter I offer activities to help with category skills, memory of new words, and opposites, as well as including activities which focus on the element of speed, which to some extent we need in order to help a conversation to run smoothly.

Spidergram

This is a vocabulary developer or lateral thinking promoter for your clients of any age. You can use it as a group activity, and in a one-to-one setting. You will be familiar with the traditional spidergram – a circle or oval 'body' drawn on a page, with eight 'legs' radiating outwards. You write a word in the middle, such as 'hobbies', 'pets' or 'clothes', and then, with your help, your client thinks of eight connected words to write at the ends of the 'legs'. You can now make these connected words into the centres of eight new spiders. The more exciting version described here might be an especially good activity to carry out at some time near Halloween.

Materials needed

- Paper (preferably A3 if your photocopier will accommodate it, as this exercise can take up a lot of room).

- Pen.

- Access to a photocopier.

- Large toy spider.

How to make your spidergram templates

A version which is deemed 'cool' by children and teenagers 'beefs up' the scary element by depicting a much more realistic spider. First, buy a plastic toy spider about 5cm across (available in toyshops). Place it on the photocopier platen, and copy it. Then recopy the result several times, with a blanked-out space in the middle of the 'spider' body to accommodate the central word. I use a small sticky label to create the space.

Procedure

Write your key word, say, 'hobbies', in the middle, leaving plenty of space round the edge. Then write a hobby at the foot of each of the spider's legs. The hobbies might be: computer games, football, pop music, dinosaurs, trains, magazines, films and holidays.

If you now draw a little spider around each of the hobbies named, you can then write at the ends of the new spider's legs. Taking 'Football' as an example, you could write: 'sport', 'goal, 'league', 'Arsenal', 'kit', 'boots', 'TV' and the name of a favourite player on this new small spider's legs.

Variations

Differently coloured little offshoot spiders make the effect less spooky but more attractive, and the hobbies would then be more easily sorted visually. It might also be easier to remember the contents of your spidergram if it is presented in this way. (Tony Buzan's 'Mind Maps' books tend to confirm this idea.)

 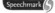

In a group setting we have used these as a front page for scrapbooks focusing on our interests, and then we found magazine pictures to illustrate each of the hobbies which we pasted inside the book – great for self- or other awareness.

If your clients don't like spiders you could draw a central flower with pointed petals instead.

One older and artistic lady I worked with drew a vase at the base of the paper, and had her different hobbies written in the flower and leaf shapes she drew emerging from the vase.

Speedy categories

This is a quick filler for ends of sessions, or as an introduction to other category work.

Materials needed

- Empty plastic drinks bottle.

- Plastic counters or stickers in a range of colours, or you can even use coloured felt tip pens.

Preparation

Place the coloured counters, stickers or pens in a large circle on the table, with the bottle in the centre.

Procedure

Take it in turns to spin the bottle. When it stops, all say the name of the nearest colour, and then the spinner has to think of as many items of that colour as they can.

Variation

To add a sense of excitement, and only for selected groups, you can try a variation where one person begins naming items while the next one is spinning the bottle for their turn.

Instead of colours round the circle, you could use stickers with letters on them, or Scrabble tiles. When the bottle stops spinning you have to think of something beginning with that particular letter. This is related to the classic 'I Spy' game, and you could also give that game a try from time to time.

Speechmark

Opposites forfeits

This is a very simple activity that should help to consolidate clients' vocabularies.

Materials needed

- Something safe to throw, for example, a Koosh ball, scrunched-up paper, or the ball that you might have made for a previous game, instructions to be found in 'DIY ball', in Chapter 5 'Conversation skills'.

- Business card blanks for the forfeit cards, which you will need to have made beforehand.

- Music will be needed if you choose to use a 'when the music stops' approach rather than a 'when you drop the ball' system.

Making the forfeit cards

Write a word on each card that has an 'opposite'. You can tailor the level of difficulty to your clients' ability levels. Easier ones might include words such as 'small', 'sad', 'quiet', 'awake', 'hate', 'black', 'old', 'no', 'rough', 'funny', 'night' and 'under'. More difficult opposites could be words such as 'generous', 'dwarf', 'tragedy', 'leisure', 'victim', 'tiptoeing' and 'sober'. Tip: you can find dozens of examples of opposite pairs on the internet.

Write the opposite words as well, on other cards – if both halves of the pair crop up during the game it does not matter at all, in fact it is an advantage, as you will be recapping.

Procedure

Your group will need to be sitting in a circle. Throw the ball from one person to the next round the circle. The first one to drop it has the forfeit of picking up a card, reading the word aloud, and giving the opposite. Or, play the music and when it stops the card is read

To begin with it is easier for the client if you select and only put out the more difficult word of the opposites pair, for example, 'narrow', so that they only have to think of 'wide', but as you progress, you can give the easier word, and they have to find the harder half of the pair. For example, give 'strange', and they must find 'familiar'.

Other uses

1 Just spread out all, or a selection, of the cards on the table, and together find the opposites pairs, in which case it isn't really a forfeit game, but is still good to play.

2 You can use the 'forfeit' approach for collective nouns. In this case write down the collective names, for example, 'shoal, flock, forest, school, gaggle, library, pride, crowd, pack, herd', and the related items, or the individual name, for example, 'fish, sheep, tree, porpoise, geese, books, lions, people, dogs (or cards), cattle'. Be a bit flexible with the responses, for example, a collective noun for 'tree' might be 'wood', 'forest' or even 'arboretum'. Some of these are fairly obscure and archaic, for example, 'a glory of goldfinches', but newer examples might include 'an album of tracks'.

3 If you are working with a group of people with Asperger's syndrome, who might use slightly old-fashioned vocabulary, you can use the same approach for learning 'street speak', providing the conventional vocabulary – 'friend', 'agreeable', 'nice person', 'concert', 'pants', 'rich', 'horrible'; and the street speak equivalents, in this case – 'mate', 'cool', 'dude', 'gig', 'keks', 'minted' and 'pants'. You may have to ask another group of clients to help you find the most current terminology, but teen magazines and slang dictionaries are useful.

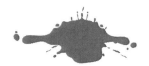

Vocabulary workbook

This is a way to work on vocabulary building in themes, with the extra value of being able to record idioms associated with each theme area. This is best done in a one-to-one session.

Materials needed

- Exercise book.
- Coloured pens or felt tips.

Procedure

Decide on some themes to be tackled. It's a good principle to go for the themes suggested by your client, usually a favourite pastime, or a school or college subject, adding some that you know they need to work on. You don't need to think of all possible themes at the start, just build them up gradually and come back and add to themes already tackled from time to time.

Allow four pages for each theme.

On the first page draw a spidergram, or mind map, with the theme word in the middle. If you are not sure about spidergrams have a look at the page on that earlier in this chapter. (Mind maps are really the same thing, but the central shape is not a spider.) This page is the place to put ideas associated with the theme. For example, if the theme happened to be 'horse riding' you would put this in the centre, adding all the generally connected ideas such as ponies, fresh air, special clothes, group, teacher, Thursday afternoons and Willow Farm. Each of these can have further connections, for example, the idea 'Willow Farm' might spawn ideas such as view, tea break, barn shelter and top field.

The second page is for all the extra, specialist vocabulary connected with the theme that you can both think of, and this would be presented in sub-themes. You can make more spidergrams for this if you like, but in this case you would need to take more pages over each major theme. For either approach, you will need to have a title and then a list of connected items. For example, the title 'Tack' would include halter, bridle, saddle and stirrups. 'Parts of the horse' would include fetlock, withers and hoof. Then there would be 'Riding gear', including jodhpurs, hard hat and boots. (I should mention that I am not actually a rider myself, but have been inspired by some of my clients!) Use different colours of pen for writing the title and content of each sub-theme; it makes it easier to remember.

The third page is for any connected idioms and, continuing with the horse-riding theme, this could include: closing the stable door after the horse has bolted; getting up on your high horse; being saddled with; and get the bit between your teeth.

Beside each idiom the client should write the agreed meaning of each idiom. This will take you from the original theme to many other areas.

The fourth page is for a quiz. You write one quiz question, for example, 'What metal things do you put your feet into when you ride?' The client adds the next question, for example, 'What is the name of my riding teacher?' Building the quiz up together in this way helps the client to 'own' their therapy. The quiz answers also call for a different kind of thinking: not starting from a central point and finding many associated ideas (as with the spidergram), which I would call 'divergent' thinking, but this time starting from an associated idea and working towards the target word, something I would call 'convergent' thinking.

Vocabulary tunnels

This is a fun way to demonstrate different types of categories. Category skills help to organise the client's already existing lexicons, and provide a place to store newly learned words. Experience suggests that the slow and deliberate action of posting word 'cars' through tubes and saying the category area arrived at should provide an image with impact that will be memorable. Car-mad boys like this activity, especially if you make it clear that the cardboard tubes are tunnels like the ones in some of the James Bond films set in the Alps!

Materials needed

- Three kitchen paper cardboard inner rolls, cut in half.

- Blu-Tack or similar.

- Small toy cars (small enough to fit through the cardboard 'tunnel'), or large marbles.

- Coloured paper: two sheets of three different colours – one of each colour left whole, and one cut into small sheets (A7 size), and then cut again into smaller strips (but big enough to write on), so you will have one whole sheet of each colour plus say 24 strips.

- Lots of sticky white labels small enough to fit on the roofs of the cars.

- Black felt tip pens, one wide, one narrow.

Preparation

This equipment can be used for many words, so it's worth spending time on making it well.

Looking first at how the game works; consider a word you might want to establish. Let's say this client likes cooking, and wants to remember the word 'colander'. This word can be defined as 'a kitchen tool used for straining, often made of metal'.

Write the word 'colander' on one of the small white labels and stick it to the top of the car or on the marble.

Think of three categories in which this word fits – let's say (1) where it's found – kitchen, (2) what it's for – straining; and (3) what it's made of – metal. (Later you can also add phonological categories.)

For each category you need one 'category tunnel'. Cover each tunnel with paper, using a different colour on each.

Write one of the category questions along the side of each tunnel. Let's say 'Where would you find it?' is on the red one. Then write 'What is it for?' along the blue one, and 'What is it made of?' along the yellow one.

Now on each small red strip of paper write down the connected place descriptors you would like to include, say sitting room, kitchen, bathroom, bedroom, garden, and so on. Write as many of these descriptors as you like because you'll use the same ones for lots of different words: you needn't use them all every time.

Now, proceed in the same way with the blue 'What is it for?' category, writing blue descriptor strips such as straining, digging, raking, heating, grating and sleeping on.

Then add the yellow 'What is it made of?' category, adding other yellow sheets saying, for example, metal, wood, fabric, plastic, pottery and china. If you have plenty of coloured paper you can add extra places, uses and materials.

Place the coloured descriptor strips on the table in their category groups, separating the groups slightly. Place the colour-coordinated tunnel in such a way that it leads towards its category group, and stick it firmly to the table with Blu-Tack.

Procedure

The client simply rolls the word car or word marble through a tunnel to the first category, 'Where would you find it?' They choose the right piece or pieces of paper from the group, and place them to the side for a moment. Now roll through the next tunnel to the next category, select the appropriate paper(s), and set them aside too, and then continue with the last tunnels. Now place the descriptors in front of the client, and place the car or marble above, and discuss the result.

One final act would be to write the word and its descriptors down (preferably in a vocabulary journal if they have one), so that you can recap next session.

Extras

You might also want to add the phonological categories such as 'Starts with …' or 'Rhymes with …', in which case just use new colours and extra tubes.

For 'Starts with …' you'll need to use the written letter rather than worrying about how to show the phonological sound.

For 'Rhymes with …' you will have to tailor-make one or two possible rhymes for each new word you are working with, and I agree that 'colander' is not an easy one to find a rhyme for, but near-rhymes might be acceptable, for instance, 'Armada' (but I'd avoid 'calendar' as it could cause confusion as the two words are so close in form).

Warning – some clients are colour blind, most commonly between red and green, so avoid using one of those colours if that condition seems likely.

Never a cross word

Crossword puzzles can be absorbing and fun, and this type will be particularly appealing as it is tailored to the client.

Use this activity one-to-one, or try it as a group activity.

Materials needed

- The crossword grid on the following page (enlarged if you like), or any other, many being available from the internet. Alternatively, just use a piece of squared paper.

- Coloured pens.

Procedure

Make a list of words connected with the client's interests, and include some long words as well as shorter ones. Suppose that they favour trains as their main interest; include words like 'footplate' and 'timetable', and add other words – 'wheels', 'ticket', 'express', 'station' and 'platform'. You might even include the names of most used stations.

Print off two versions of the grid – you will need one to fill in yourself, to make the thing work, and another for your client.

For your grid: write the longest word in the centre, either horizontally or vertically, and line up a long word going the opposite way, linking them together by a mutual letter, preferably fairly centrally – for example, there is a *t* near the centres of the words 'footplate' and 'timetable'. Add other words and blank out (scribble in) some squares as necessary to make each word link only at the points you have decided. In principle it's best to place the longer words first, adding shorter ones as fillers afterwards. If you are stuck for a link then just leave a few squares blank – we are not trying to become *Times'* crossword writers! You can always make a second puzzle including the words you left out last time.

Number the words.

For your client's grid: to make the equivalent version for your client you need to blank out the same squares as those in the original and, also in the same way as the original, you need to number the squares where the client will write the words. Photocopy this as a spare.

Now you need to write the clues, numbered of course to correspond to the words on your grid. Take care over the level of difficulty of the clues and the type, because you need to reinforce the classification of words to fit in with your therapy. If, for example, you have been working on phonological categories you would include as many as possible of these as parts of clues. For example, 'They rhyme with snails, and a train goes along on them'. Present these on the same sheet of paper as the client's grid. Photocopy again – some clients dislike making a mistake and might need a fresh copy.

If they feel able, your clients might like to try inventing their own crossword puzzles for each other, or to place in a college magazine.

Here's one I made earlier...

Category sleuths

This is another game to help clients understand the way in which words are classified into categories. I admit that it is a bit fiddly to make, but I think you will find the end result well worthwhile. You can use it as a group game or in a one-to-one setting. The aim is to elicit questions from your clients, who try to 'home in on' the right word by progressively narrowing down from a broad category to finer and finer definitions.

Materials needed

- The tiles from a defunct Scrabble game. You need the plastic rather than the wooden type, because you are going to tuck a 5p coin in the hollow under one of the tiles. You don't need a complete set of the tiles, as you are going to change the fronts.

- A box to keep the tiles in.

- Widgit or Clipart symbols printed out in a small size. You will need nouns, and think in terms of these sorts of categories: sports, furniture, toys, weather, plants, foods, office, kitchen and animals.

- Also subdivide your categories if you can, so that within the 'sports' category you might have racquet sports, team games, sport clothes, and so on.

- In the 'animals' category you might have examples in these types: zoo animals, farm animals and pets. Alternatively, or in addition, you could use examples from the ordering of taxonomy, so that you would have insects, birds, mammals, reptiles, fish, amphibians, and so on.

- Try to have other category types included too, for example, made of metal, red, edible or roundish. Words will appear in more than one category, which is very useful as this then helps participants to narrow down their choices.

- Glue.

- A 5p coin (or a small counter would be fine).

Procedure

Decide on how many tiles you are going to use. It's probably best to start with just a few – you can always build up to a greater number as you go on. Select a few tiles from, say, three main categories. Put these out on the table, hiding the coin or counter underneath one tile, and remember where you have hidden it!

You will have to demonstrate at first, arranging and role playing the questioner as well as the person who answers. This might be the pattern of questions and answers:

Q. Is it under an animal?

A. Yes.

So you now clear away all the non-animal pictures.

    Q. Does it have four legs?

    A. No.

So you clear away all those with four legs, and might now be left with a green parrot, a goldfish, an orange butterfly, a green caterpillar, a person dressed in orange and a green beetle. Now the questioner must think of the best way to narrow down, so could either go for colour, for example:

    Q. Is it green?

or go for another attribute, for example:

    Q. Can it fly?

And so on! Now you can see why it's important to have as many cross-category pictures as possible. What you are trying to avoid is the one-tile approach; 'Is it under the caterpillar?', 'No'; 'Is it under the ice-cream?', 'No'. This will take forever, and will not result in category learning.

Once the correct tile has been chosen that person (the winner) takes the task of hiding the coin (with the others turning away).

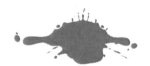

Speechmark

Egg timer words

Here is a vocabulary game to help clients make words at speed. Those who read fairly easily will be able to play this game against the egg timer, but a different version can be played if the clients have more difficulty in reading, or lack confidence in this area. It can be great fun, but some clients might find it a bit panic-inducing, or too competitive, so tread carefully.

You can use it as a group game or in a one-to-one setting.

Materials needed

- The tiles from a defunct Scrabble game. It isn't essential to have a complete set of tiles, but of course if you have a 'Q' you'll need to have at least one 'U' in the set.

- A box to keep the tiles in.

- An egg timer. A kitchen egg timer lasts for three minutes, but if you feel your clients might need to work at a slower pace, a kitchen 'pinger' is ideal for setting longer timings.

Procedure

Deal out 20 tiles each, letter side down.

When you turn over the egg timer or start the kitchen pinger and say 'Go!', everyone turns over their tiles and tries to make as many words, of three or more letters, as they can before the time is up. The winner is the person who has used up the greatest number of tiles in real (not invented) words. Proper nouns are usually disallowed, although there are times when you might bend this rule.

Other ideas to help with vocabulary development

Please see also:

1 For adjectives, try 'Life of Riley' in Chapter 7 'Lateral thinking'.

2 'Alternative odd one out', also in Chapter 7 'Lateral thinking'.

3 As a development of category skills, 'Remembering in threes' in Chapter 8 'Memory'.

 Speechmark

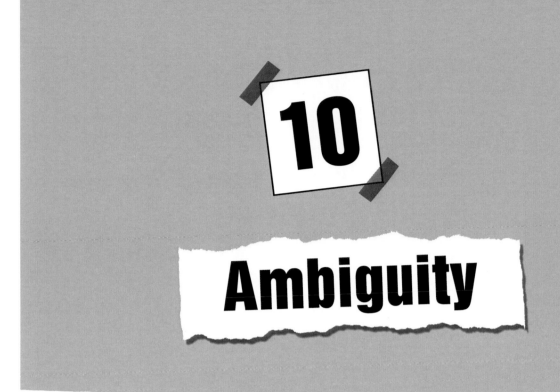

10

Ambiguity

How confusing the following phrases could be to people who take the unintended meaning of such commonly seen public notices:

Fine for parking here – does that mean it's OK to park here, or that you will get a parking ticket?

Cats' eyes removed in next stretch – something for the vet to do, or roadworks ahead?

Baby changing room – change nappies here, or swap your baby for another one?

In our language a word, a saying, a proverb or a slang expression can mean two (or more) things at the same time. For most of us, everyday expressions such as 'Hang on a moment', or 'Pull your socks up' are immediately understandable, but they can be puzzling to literal thinkers.

In particular, for those with an autism spectrum disorder this type of language can be bewildering and distressing, and could lead to many misunderstandings or isolation in social situations.

I offer my understanding of some of the terminology used to describe ambiguous language:

Figurative language is an overarching term meaning language that is enhanced by idioms, metaphors, similes, proverbs, and so on.

Idioms are forms of language that are invented, agreed, dispersed and understood by speakers of a particular language. They are forms of expression where the meaning is not predictable from the individual words, for example, 'It cost me an arm and a leg'. They have often come originally from a working or a sporting context, for example, 'He shut the stable door after the horse had bolted', or 'A sticky wicket'.

A *metaphor* is a word or phrase which, if taken literally, would be incorrect when applied to the object being described, for example, 'Life is a journey' and 'All the world's a stage' (Shakespeare).

There are two special types of figurative language associated with metaphor, which often confuse our clients. In 'metonymy', the literal is replaced by something associated with it, for example, 'Can I have another cup?' when you are asking for a cup of tea, or 'Give me your ears please', to get attention in class. There is also 'synecdoche', which replaces something either with a part of the something, or the whole class to which the something belongs. For instance, 'give her a hand, Bob', or 'the Crown spoke to the prime minister'.

A *simile* is a phrase which compares one thing with another of a different kind, and usually contains the word 'like' or 'as'. For example, 'Life is rather like a tin of sardines: we're all looking for the key' (Alan Bennett).

A *proverb* is a short, pithy, often traditional saying which expresses something obvious, true, or profound: 'Look after the pennies and the pounds will look after themselves'.

A *pun* is a play on words, where the words sound alike but have different meanings. They are humorous in a groan-making way! (I have to admit that once they have been taken apart and explained to a client they may become rather less amusing!)

You don't really need to know much more than that to work with the speech-based activities in this chapter, but there is also a section on non-verbal ambiguity.

'Lovely weather', a comment said with a glum face, could be confusing because, in addition to spoken ambiguities, there are all the subtleties of mismatches between facial expression, tone of voice and the actual words spoken, which form the basis of sarcasm and other subliminal messages. It may take a good deal of therapy before some clients will begin to understand that meanings often need to be taken from the speaker's face rather than the words.

Having struggled with various schemes to begin to tackle the large and difficult area of ambiguity for clients with an autism spectrum disorder, I would suggest that ambiguous pictures are a key to introducing the initial concept. Clients usually find these pictures interesting and informative, so this chapter begins with an activity based on that. I hope you enjoy using these games and activities designed to fight confusion.

Visual ambiguities activity

I have found that an excellent way to prepare clients for learning that words can mean more than one thing is to begin with pictures that mean two things. This activity is suitable for a small group.

I think a small explanation of the way in which I understand the terms 'optical illusion' and 'ambiguous image' might be useful.

Optical illusions: these are images that trick or tease the eye, making you think that one thing is correct when in fact another is. Have you ever gazed at an image of swirly concentric circles that soon appear to be moving? Have you seen that picture of two lines which are identical except that one has outward-pointing 'arrows' on both ends, and the other has inward-pointing ones, so that the 'outward pointer' seems to be longer? These are both examples of optical illusion.

Visual ambiguities: these are images that show two things at once – the face-to-face profiles which form the shape of a goblet in the space between them, or the head of a horse that can be drawn in such a way as to also look like the whole body of a seal (the ears of the horse become the tail of the seal).

Materials needed

The easiest way to gather images for this activity used to be to look at the illustrations in the Yellow Pages (eg they used a picture of a banana skin for the section on insurance, and one of an ice lolly for loans – 'Need some Lolly?') but, alas, there are few of these images in the new directories, so if you have any of the old variety do hang on to them!

Other sources are psychology books with a section on visual processing – you will tend to find the classic image of a woman who can be seen either as young or old, and the face-to-face profiles of two people, which is at the same time one person's full face.

Another source is a book about the artist Escher who created images such as repeat patterns of birds with the intervening spaces forming other birds, or fish, or fields. You should be able to borrow this book from a library, or his images are also available as inexpensive postcards.

Also keep an eye on magazine and newspaper adverts; very many of them are based on visual ambiguities.

There are also some lovely coffee-table books of images of optical illusions and ambiguous images. These are expensive, but you can borrow them from libraries, or maybe ask for one for a present!

Procedure

Photocopy any images that copyright permits, cut out magazine adverts, and put them into plastic pockets to protect them. (This also makes the images easier to store in a file.) It is a good idea to have several images to use at the same time, because I have found that this work is really interesting for the clients, and they all want to look at the pictures simultaneously.

Hand out images to the group members, or pass the book round, and ask them to say what they see. If they cannot visualise one of the images, you may find that another client can, but that they in turn cannot see the one that the first client saw. Have them explain to each other what they can see, or guide them through the visualisation process yourself. You may have to redraw elements of the image to make it really clear.

After you have spent some time looking at the images and discussing them, it is good to make the point that just as pictures can mean two things, so can individual words. Give examples of this, for example, each of the words 'run', 'train' and 'mobile' has at least two different meanings. At your next session you could recap on a few pictures, and the idea of individual word ambiguity, and then begin to work towards whole phrase ambiguity – for example, 'Pull your socks up'. If you look on the National Autistic Society's website (www. nas.org.uk) you will find a long list of such idioms, or just key in 'Idioms' to the internet and you will find dozens of examples.

You may also be able to start work on the simplest pun-based jokes at this point, in which case please see the 'Save your cracker jokes' activity in this chapter.

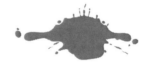

 Speechmark

Body idioms

This is a group activity finishing up with an image that is made with your clients actually there with you – so not strictly 'made earlier'. It is designed to promote understanding of idiom, and is good fun to do, but you need to have a brave (and still) soul who is prepared to be drawn round!

Materials needed

- Very large piece of paper, approximately 2m x 600mm – two lengths of lining wallpaper taped together along the length would be fine.

- Or, a large blackboard would do, if it is the right height from the floor and large enough to contain the 'template person'.

- Wide and narrow water-based felt tips or board chalk.

Procedure

Draw round your person (or you could just draw a person shape if participants are too shy).

Together think of all the sayings you can that are connected with the body.

Write them on the relevant part.

You will probably come up with sayings such as: 'head for heights'; 'made my hair stand on end'; 'making eyes at'; 'I'm all ears'; 'don't bite my head off'; 'chip on their shoulder'; 'lend a hand'; 'green fingers'; 'pain in the neck'; 'heart in the right place'; 'butterflies in my tummy'; 'they've got guts'; 'sitting on their bottom all day'; 'legless'; 'feet on the floor'; 'treading on someone's toes'; 'Achilles heel'. There must be dozens more of these – the best ones will be those the clients think of themselves.

As the clients add each saying, discuss the ambiguity and the way it is used, and request that they use them in a sentence or two, so that they become familiar.

Variations

You can also draw a 'wardrobe' – it's amazing how many expressions are based on clothes. Examples include: 'pull your socks up'; 'down at heel'; 'bore the pants off'; 'to pocket something'; 'to skirt round'; 'cloak and dagger'; 'keep it under your hat'.

Save your cracker jokes

Most cracker jokes are based on puns and idioms: forms of ambiguity that are sometimes difficult for people on the autism spectrum to understand.

Humour, even the corny pun, adds to enjoyment of life, and I feel a need to open the door of this enjoyable part of life to the clients. I have found that it is possible to dismantle these simple jokes, explain them step by step, and then put them back together again, thereby making them accessible and enjoyable for all. Many young people with Asperger's syndrome are motivated by this work. It is best not to introduce this until some preparation has taken place through the 'Visual ambiguities' activity, and perhaps other work on idiom.

The idea (and in my experience this does work) is that as you examine more and more pun-type jokes the clients will begin to understand the system, and start to enjoy them on their own. The additional benefits are that they should then have a few jokes up their sleeves for social occasions; be more open to understanding other people's puns that crop up in conversation; and may also have widened their vocabulary and knowledge of idiom.

Beware: for some reason the most groan-making jokes are the ones that seem to be most easily remembered, and will be re-quoted at you long afterwards!

Materials needed

- As many cracker jokes as you can possibly get. I've found that within a brand of cracker they tend to repeat the same jokes, so it is a good idea to ask your friends and family to save their cracker jokes too so that you stand more chance of acquiring many different jokes. You can, of course, find books of puns as an alternative source.

- A4 paper.

- Glue.

- Access to photocopier.

Procedure

Carefully pick out the jokes you are going to work with; you are looking for the ones with obvious puns and idioms.

Stick the jokes, well spaced out, on pieces of A4, and make photocopies for each group member.

The core of the work is to find the word or idiomatic phrase that means two things, the 'double entendre'.

For example, look at this old joke: Patient: 'Doctor, Doctor, I feel like a pair of curtains'. Doctor: 'Well pull yourself together then'. It is the words 'pull yourself together' which mean two things; in one sense we take the words literally, as in pulling curtains, and in the other sense we mean 'take control of your behaviour'. This double meaning is the key to the joke, and the reason for its inaccessibility to many people on the autism spectrum. They tend to go for the literal meaning only, so miss out on the duality of meaning – the pun is lost. Here you will have to explain the idiomatic meaning and recap the other, literal one, and then retell the joke.

What about another old one: 'My dog's got no nose'; 'How does he smell then?'; 'Terrible'. Here the pun is with the word 'smell'. This is an easier one to explain as no idioms are involved, just two meanings of the one word.

Once you have explained the procedure about finding the pun word using a few of the jokes, you can ask one of the other group members to pick out the next pun in the same way.

This work was so popular with our group that they decided to collate their favourites into a little book. We photocopied just four duplex A4 sheets of jokes and a front and back cover, folded and stapled them together, and then sold the booklet at our Christmas market in aid of our local branch of the National Autistic Society in Stroud. They sent us a lovely thank-you letter, which in turn further raised the self-esteem of the group members.

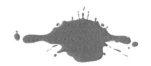

Newspaper headlines

This is an activity that will further the clients' work on ambiguity, and should be a source of humour.

Materials needed

Newspapers. Tabloids seem to be best at producing both intentional and unintentional puns. Local papers are also good sources.

Procedure

Present the punning headlines on the list offered here one at a time, and work out together which is the ambiguous word in each headline.

Look through these examples before you present them to your group, and avoid any that you feel are inappropriate. However, if you use these in a talk, as a way of demonstrating to staff the meaning of 'ambiguous phrases', you will probably find, as I have, that your audience finds all the examples very funny (but they do distract them slightly from attending to the rest of the talk, so it is wise to give these as handouts at the end of the talk, or at a break).

Suggested headlines to get you started:

Drunk Gets Nine Months in Violin Case

Hospitals are Sued by Seven Foot Doctors

Panda Mating Fails; Vet Takes Over

Squad Helps Dog Bite Victim

Shot Off Woman's Leg Helps Golfer to Victory

Enraged Cow Injures Farmer with Axe

Juvenile Court to Try Shooting Defendant

Stolen Painting Found by Tree

Two Sisters Reunited After Fifteen Years in Checkout Counter

Miners Refuse to Work After Death

Red Tape Holds Up New Bridge

Man Struck by Lightening Faces Battery Charge

Kids Make Nutritious Snacks

Sex Education Delayed, Teachers Request Training

Include Your Children When Baking Cookies

Head Seeks Arms

Now go through the papers you have brought in, and see if anyone can find any new puns.

If you listen to *The News Quiz* on Radio 4 you will hear a few more examples each week.

These following unintentional puns are notices rather than headlines – but just as ambiguous!

Eye Drops Off Shelf

Trousers Down by 50 Per Cent

See if your group can add any that they may have come across, or set this as a task for the following week.

Idiom journals

This is a long-term, ongoing activity for individuals who find it difficult to understand and remember idiomatic language: sayings, expressions or metaphors. Even proverbs could be included here. Making a journal is useful as it is a way to note things down until they can be discussed; a record of the meanings; provides an interesting way to look at how much has been learned, and can act as an awareness tool. You will probably find that idioms are written down more frequently as time goes on, because your client is noticing them more.

Have a look at the 'Vocabulary workbook' in Chapter 9 'Vocabulary' for a way of integrating idiom work with vocabulary development.

Materials needed

- A notebook or an exercise book divided into several sections – for example, home, weather, travel, cookery and any topics that the client works with or studies, such as gardening, farming, seamanship or mending.

- If the client has access to their computer from your clinic, or brings their laptop, you could do all this more easily via word processing as then it is easier to change things, and add extras.

Procedure

Together think of all the sayings you can that are connected with each topic. Write each example in the appropriate section and add alongside it the meaning and the date you discussed it.

After the session the client should take their book with them and add more examples as they occur to them, especially those that crop up while they are doing the connected activity, or those that are actually said to them. If they feel that they can ask the meaning they should add that at the time, otherwise they can bring it to the next session for discussion.

The reason for adding the dates is that you can decide together the length of time after which to retest them – you might want to review after a week, a month or a term.

Encourage the client to practise using the idiomatic phrase in a sentence. Set up a role play for this so that the saying will be within a context. Even if the client doesn't use the phrase outside of the clinic it is a useful way to learn and 'fix' the meaning.

Other activities to help with understanding ambiguity

Please see also:

1 The 'Other uses' section of 'Opposites forfeits' in Chapter 9 'Vocabulary'.

2 'Vocabulary workbook', also in Chapter 9 'Vocabulary'.

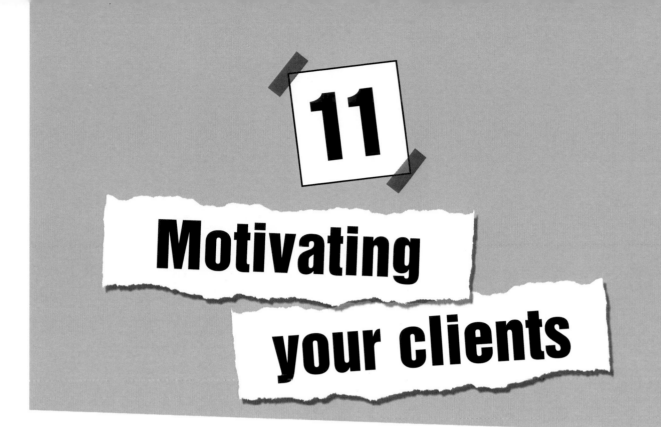

Motivating your clients

No matter how much fun your sessions are, or how much your clients feel they are learning, or how interested they have been, there may come a point when they need a new challenge, or another way of boosting their motivation.

Sometimes we have to acknowledge that a break from therapy is needed, but first it might be worth considering a small change, or adding a new element to the therapy to get things going again. Even if you decide to discontinue the therapy for the time being it is important to end the period of therapy on a winning, positive note, so that if they return for further therapy ,they won't remember the last session as being boring.

All of the games throughout this book are designed to be motivating, because they should be different from regular forms of therapy, and fun as well as informative. In this chapter, however, there are some extras, outside of the main scope of your therapy – a game to intrigue adults, another one to promote cooperation between children, one just generally to have everyone laughing, and one to refresh the attention spans of clients jaded by too much work.

Cooperation tin

A useful activity early in the life of a SLT group for children. It illustrates the benefits of working with rather than against each other! The participants need to be roughly of equal strengths. The making of this item seems fiddly, but it is worth taking the time to produce something sturdy.

Materials needed

- A round biscuit tin, approx 20cm in diameter
- Three 2m lengths of strong nylon cord.
- Six rubber grommets, large enough for the cord to pass through.
- Drill.
- Treats!

Brawn needed

Drill six equally spaced holes around the side of the tin, about halfway down the side, the diameter of the inner core of the grommets.

Completing the tin

Fit the grommets into the holes in the tin. Thread the cords through the grommets and then tie them together in the middle. Tie knots in the outer ends of the cords to form 'handles'.

Procedure

Sit the participants in a circle on the floor, or round a table, with the tin in the centre.

Each person should hold a rope.

Place six, preferably wrapped, treats in the tin – in a bag is a hygienic idea – and make clear that the clients may only take one treat, and that they may only do so when the tin touches them. (If your group has challenging behaviour, you may need to restrict the number in the tin to one treat at a time and then top up after each turn.)

They are now allowed to pull on the ropes, but they will soon find that the tin will only touch someone if everyone allows it, that is, five people must slacken their ropes while one person pulls. In theory at least, they will begin to see that taking turns at receiving the treat is good for everyone.

Try to emphasise that cooperation is a good thing, even if it seems that you have to wait a long time before you get a treat.

This activity also provides a good analogy for conversational turn taking – if you hog the conversation you will end up with a lot of unhappy listeners. Make this point very clearly, and invite discussion about it.

Cooperation balloons

This is a great activity that is really an adapted classic party game. It's good fun perhaps as an end-of-term game, or at any time to add to work on correct conversational distance. A biggish group of eight clients is ideal, although it can be done with four. The game helps to establish a mood of cooperation and fun, encourages practice in greetings and social chat, and illustrates the benefits of working with a partner. The partners need to be of roughly equal height.

Materials needed

- Balloons.
- Pin.
- Wide, soft felt tips.

Getting started

The first thing to establish is whether any of the participants have a fear of balloons! Quite often people on the autism spectrum worry that a balloon will explode in their face. One thing to try as a demonstration is the 'controlled pop' – a way in which they can be in charge of a gentle explosion. All you need to do is to blow up an extra balloon, a little softer than its full capacity, and show the clients how to take the pin, and gently stick it into the wrinkled, slightly thicker area around the knot. The balloon will not explode loudly, but will merely puff and deflate. Really. Try it on your own first if you are not convinced! Once this has been done the clients tend to feel that they have control over the balloons, and are therefore not worried about them any more.

Now ask everyone to blow up a balloon, again not too hard.

They should draw a face on each balloon with the soft felt tips.

Procedure

In the original party games the balloon is placed between the foreheads of the partners, and the pairs race sideways, like a racing crab, or else the balloon is passed from one person to the next between the knees. However, for people with an ASD such closeness can be intolerable. In this humorous 'buffered contact' version, the balloon is sandwiched between the shoulders of two clients who are standing side by side with the balloon's drawn-on face looking forward. Two pairs of clients with their sandwiched balloons stand opposite each other, at a distance, and then carefully walk towards each other so that the balloon faces eventually reach conversational distance from each other. If the balloons are still in place by the time the couples meet, they can proceed to the next stage.

Now the clients make their balloons have a conversation with one another, that is, the clients talk in an animated way that causes their shoulders (and therefore the balloons) to shift about. The couple who first let their balloon drop are out. They will find that the funnier the chat the more likely the balloons are to fall. Another method of making the opposite couple drop their balloon is to make comments about something that is either high up, or on the floor. Moving about will risk losing the shoulder-to-shoulder pressure, and so dropping the balloon.

The last ones with a balloon are the winners.

Butterfly game

This is a fun game for any client, but particularly those with short attention spans ('butterfly minds'), or those whose targets you are trying to disguise rather than 'turn them off' therapy.

Materials needed

- You need a way of choosing a number. Either use a dice (bought, or home made out of sponge as per 'Question dice' in Chapter 5 on conversation skills), or – perhaps a more interesting and active idea – spin an empty plastic bottle, which ends up pointing at a numbered sticker applied to the table.

- Several pre-arranged activities (six if you are using an ordinary dice). Some of these will be activities used for that client's specific targets – they could be some facial expression cards to copy; some 'find the difference' cards to work out; some sequence cards; and maybe a category heading (sports or hobbies for your client to respond to). Other, 'relief', activities could be some bubble-blow, some tiddlywinks to ping into a saucer, or two or three balls, to try juggling.

- Paper carrier bags or shoeboxes, preferably plain coloured, to hide the activities in, and some stickers to apply to them to give the number corresponding to the dice or spin-a-bottle numbers.

Procedure

Simply roll the dice or spin the bottle, check the number, and carry out the corresponding activity. Just do one card from the corresponding box, or one blow of the bubbles, for example, and don't take too long at each task.

My advice is to be cheery but firm from the start about sticking to the activity your client arrives at when they spin or throw, otherwise there is a possibility that they will always engineer things to be able to carry out their favourite one!

Palindromes

This is an activity that will appeal to clients who are already interested in language and writing, or who need to find some light-heartedness in communication. They will be fascinated to see how a sentence can be read forwards or backwards, and can have fun working out established ones, like those listed, or even have a go at making up their own. Use this as a group activity, or try it one-to-one. The idea of the activity is to promote interest in words in general.

Materials needed
• Paper and pens.

Procedure

Write one palindrome on a sheet of paper for each client, and ask them if they can see anything odd about it. Once they have worked it out, give them another and another, until you can let them see the whole list.

Madam I'm Adam

I saw desserts: I'd no lemons, alas no melon. Distressed was I.

Live not on evil

Pull up if I pull up

Step on no pets

Was it a rat I saw

Ma is a nun as I am

Never odd or even

We panic in a pew

Ample help Ma

Desserts I stressed

Night, fifth gin

A man a plan a canal Panama!

Sums are not set as a test on Erasmus

Niagara, o roar again!

If they feel able, your clients might like to try inventing their own palindromes. If so, it is worthwhile looking back at the examples given, and working out which is the central letter, demonstrating that the word breaks on each side of the centre need not be the same, and that punctuation is not counted. It is also useful to have a list of some single palindromic words handy. These are words such as 'deed', 'toot', 'minim', 'level', 'civic', 'madam', 'pip', 'pop', 'rotor', 'radar', 'eye', 'nun', and 'racecar'. They can form the middle word, or could be either side of the centre, to form the simplest type of palindrome, for example, a driving instructor one: 'Toot madam, toot', or 'Level, Anna, level'.

Projects

Showing off their 'special interests' can often revive therapy that has focused on an area of work for longer than the client can manage. This activity will vary according to your client — one may be interested in trains, while another may like film scripts, gardens, the history of chocolate, or fashions.

The starting point for an activity leads to other, related topics; one older student we worked with was interested in beer and pubs so we guided him to the idea of the brewing process and its history rather than just listing pubs he liked to visit.

Some clients are more able, and will be able to collect items for their project themselves, while others will need support.

Materials needed

- A scrapbook with a cover that can be decorated. Alternatively, clients could use a ringbinder and plastic polypockets, but this is a more expensive option.

- As many leaflets, pictures from the internet and photos about the chosen topic as possible. The client may need to write to manufacturers (eg to Thorntons or Green and Black's, to obtain leaflets about chocolate making).

- Information about the topic – from the internet if necessary, but the client's own experiences are even better.

Procedure

The client should spend some time arranging the leaflets in a good order, such that they can add text to their project in a coherent way, developing their ideas into a pleasant end product that they will be pleased to show.

If there are going to be enough spare pages it is wise to leave a few blank, so that even after sticking in their leaflets and text they would still be able to add further material. If they are using the ringbinder option it is much easier to insert extra items.

Extension to the project

If they feel able, your clients might like to aim towards giving a short talk about their project – either to their SLT group, or to a larger audience.

Other ideas for motivating your clients

Please see also:

1 'Paint splotch predictions' in Chapter 2 'Self-awareness and self-esteem'.

2 'Soap box' in Chapter 4 'Listening skills'.

3 'Friendship consequences' in Chapter 13 'Friendships and relationships'.

4 'Customised Jenga' in Chapter 14 'End-of-course and recap games'.

5 'Life of Riley' in Chapter 7 'Lateral thinking'.

6 'Gesture darts' in Chapter 12 'Body language'.

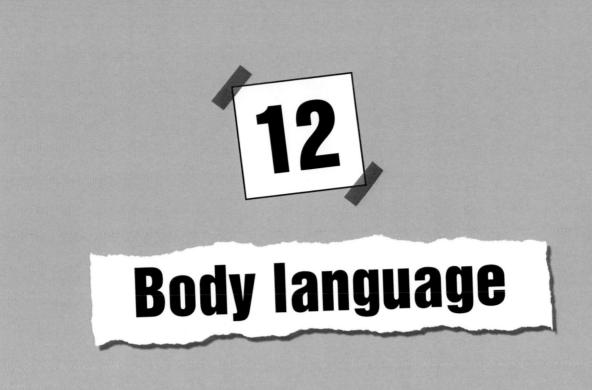

12

Body language

Have you ever watched films or programmes on TV that show body language so clearly that words are not needed? The French mime expert Marcel Marceau miming how to clean a window; Rowan Atkinson acting 'Mr Bean', and even some children's cartoons such as *Pingu* all demonstrate the power of body language. Some theorists state that as much as 60 per cent or more of our communication is transmitted by body language (and other non-verbal communication, such as tone of voice, may contribute even more).

To demonstrate to yourself how much you use body language, try, as if you were talking to a small child, to describe the movement of a wind turbine, but without moving your arms; or talk about the extreme quietness of a bat's squeak, but without wrinkling up the corners of your eyes.

Some clients have great difficulty with body language – they may not notice others using it; not understand the link between emotion and facial expression or body language; or not be able to use it accurately themselves to enhance their spoken words or to convey an emotion.

This chapter attempts to address the problem of how to help these clients. Good humour and a little exaggeration are put to use sometimes, and the activities are designed to meet the needs of clients of different ages.

Eye instruct you

This is a group game for young children to encourage eye contact, and can be stretched to become a memory game too. It is useful for a quick 'filler' activity and takes virtually no preparation.

Materials needed

- One pair of spectacle frames (old sunglasses with the lenses pushed out are fine), or you can use your hands: form circles with your index fingers and thumbs, and put them over your eyes.

- One foam or Koosh ball, or use the DIY ball mentioned in Chapter 5 on conversation skills (or even just scrunched-up paper if you're feeling really short of budget and/or time).

Procedure

One person (any of the clients, or the therapist) wears the glasses. Another person has the ball.

Try to make it clear that everybody must carefully watch the person wearing the glasses, otherwise they won't know where to throw the ball.

The person wearing the glasses indicates *with their eyes only* another person in the group to whom the ball must be thrown, and then the ball is thrown.

Now a new person has the glasses, and you start again.

Variation

You can extend this by looking at two people, so the catcher throws to one person, who then throws to the second one. This involves everyone in close watching and remembering.

Gesture darts

If you ever work with a group of disaffected teenage boys with poor body language, this is one activity to pounce on as, in my experience, it will pass the 'coolness' test! For part of the time it is an activity which requires the participants to express and instruct; for the rest of the time there is some 'test piloting' to be done; a little writing (but you can help); and some posture and gesture work.

Be warned — it is almost inevitable that you will get some rude gestures as offerings to the game. My advice is to say at the start that you already know these and that they are too easy. If they do crop up again, just acknowledge, and pass swiftly on.

As far as safety is concerned, I have never had a problem with this, although you could make sure that the darts are softened slightly, by poking them down on to the table to crumple the points just a little. You should also be clear that the darts must be aimed at the chest of the person, or stand up and aim for the feet. If you are still worried, then this activity is not for you.

Materials needed

• Paper and pens.

Procedure

Provide an example of a folded paper dart. Keep it simple, so that the clients have a chance to offer their improved versions. Encourage some of the clients to instruct and demonstrate their dart folding techniques. Stand side by side in a line at the end of the room and practise the dart throwing technique. Have a few test runs to see which darts are the best fliers. Be careful on the congratulations front, and try to think of plus points for all the designs, for example, 'long flier', 'nice and steady', 'good short flight for working round a table', 'nice big space to write on' or 'interesting new design'. It is important to be generous in your praise if the participants are boys, because they seem to regard engineering- and pilot-related activities as a sign of their manliness for some reason!

Now ask the clients to write on their darts the gesture or posture that they want another person to perform. These could be whole body language signals such as 'I'm going to sneeze', 'I'm really tired', 'My stomach aches', 'I'm hitching a lift' or 'I've hurt my ankle'; or they could be simpler instructions, for example, 'wave', 'nod', 'stick out your tongue' or 'shrug your shoulders'. They could even be instructions for the recipient to demonstrate a Signalong or Makaton sign.

Half of the clients line up at one end of the room, and half face them at the other end. Ask all but one of the clients to put the darts down for a moment, while the other one throws their dart towards the feet of someone at the other end of the room. That person picks up the dart, silently reads the instruction, and performs the gesture or posture, and then throws the dart back to someone else (not the originator) at the first end of the room, who must do likewise. Once everyone has had a go, the originator reads the instruction aloud, and all do the gesture together. Now move on to the next dart, and so on until all darts have been thrown and examined by all.

If you worry that they are all going to just chuck them anywhere the best solution is to keep the darts by you, handing them out one at a time when the previous one has been tried and discussed.

Speechmark

Where am I looking?

A game to encourage eye contact without the pressure of meeting each other's gaze. It is a good opportunity, also, to practise sign language. It is suitable for a group of three or four of any age, depending on which items you choose to use.

Materials needed

- Small objects (eg cup, pen, ball and food items).
- Photo cards, preferably of single nouns.

Procedure

The therapist shows the clients each object or photo card and makes sure that they know the name or sign for it.

The items are placed around the room allowing the clients to watch. It is sensible, at least to start with, to space the items as widely apart as possible. Later, as the clients improve at looking at the direction of your gaze, you can bring the items closer together.

The therapist asks, 'What am I looking at?' with a steady gaze at one item; the clients must guess, and name or sign it. Do this for each item, and then add some new items or images.

When the clients are ready they themselves can take turns to have a go at this.

Clairvoyance

Not real clairvoyance of course, but definitely a form of mind reading! This activity promotes understanding of facial expressions, and of other people's points of view, and is useful for a group of fairly able clients with Asperger's syndrome. There are already boxes of photo cards on the market, but in this version the accompanying newspaper article has a role to play. Also, these pictures can be written on, and will have been selected by the clients themselves.

Materials needed

- Clear pictures of individuals, preferably showing facial expression, gesture and particular kinds of clothing that give them a bit of character. Extra clues will come from the context of the photo: country scene, war zone, fashion shoot, office, and so on. Good sources for photos are magazines, colour supplements and newspapers (but avoid 'page 3' type pictures as they will cause so much diversion that you might as well give up the session!).

- Scissors (left- and right-handed).

- Paper and glue.

- Pens.

- Post-it notes.

How to be clairvoyant!

Each group member cuts out their chosen picture of a person. No one should read the connected article, as then they are not being clairvoyant! Mark both the picture and the article with an identifying number or squiggle, and pass to the group leader for secure keeping. Now guess four things about the picture:

What could their name be?

What are they thinking?

What are their plans?

What are they about to say?

Each group member takes a picture (preferably not the one they previously selected and cut out), sticks a Post-it note on to it with their interpretation, and then passes it on to a neighbour for a different interpretation.

The moment of truth

Now you or your client reads the original accompanying article, to see how close the client's ideas were to the truth.

Variation

If the clients might be tempted to peep at the article, you would have to resort to cutting the pictures out yourself beforehand. Again, it's wise to make sure you know which article goes with which picture.

Dicing with your emotions

This is a useful and fun activity, particularly for a group of students with an ASD. You can use it as a five-minute 'filler' or extend it into two 20-minute exercises.

Materials needed

- Mirror (preferably either a proper therapy mirror, with good reflective qualities but unbreakable, or a large one that is fixed to the wall).

- Two or more sponge or polystyrene cubes approximately 10cm in size, either from a toyshop, or home made out of sponge as per 'Question dice' in Chapter 5 'Conversation skills'.

- Simple images of facial expressions stuck on to sticky labels. You can use Widgit symbols for these, or Clipart pictures, or you can do your own artwork; or simply write the emotions on the sides of the cubes, if your clients are readers.

Completing the dice

Buy or make at least two cubes, writing the easier expressions on one and more subtle ones on the other. (While you are at the making stage you could add another one which you might need later, for 'Variation 2'. This one needs to show the questions suggested there.)

Easier examples: 'happy', 'sad', 'angry', 'surprised', 'disgusted' and 'scared'.

Subtle: 'confused', 'worried', 'shocked', 'unsure', 'tired', 'disappointed', 'content', 'amused', 'hopeful', 'exhausted', 'interested' and 'determined' (I'd avoid 'bored'!)

Procedure

Each member of the group takes a turn to roll the cube with the simple expressions, and just copies the expression on the dice. They can check in a mirror to make sure that they are making the face they intended.

Repeat the process using the more complicated 'subtle' expressions.

Repeat, but this time hide the dice from the others, who must guess the expression being shown. The person who successfully guesses the expression then rolls the dice.

Now each person tries rolling both dice at the same time. They make one 'face', and then the other one, for the others to guess.

Variations

Variation 1. Two people each have a dice; they roll, and make the face, then, by looking at each other (not each other's dice), swap facial expressions, and then check on the dice to see if they have made the right face.

 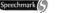

Variation 2. Add and roll another dice which shows the following questions and instructions:

> *Which gestures and postures go with …?*
>
> *What could be another word for this emotion …?*
>
> *What might I say when I feel …?*
>
> *How do I sound when I feel …?*
>
> *Count up to 10 as if you feel …*
>
> *Say the days of the week as if you feel …*

The client rolls this question dice at the same time as one of the emotions dice. They make the facial expression shown and then follow the question or instruction, for instance:

You might roll 'sad', and then, supposing that on the question dice you have rolled 'Which gestures and postures go with …?', you would droop your head, sag your shoulders, and so on.

Or if you've rolled 'angry' with "What could be another word for this emotion …?', you might say 'furious', 'cross', 'grumpy', and so on.

Or if you have rolled 'happy' with 'What might I say when I feel …?', you might say 'Yes! Hooray! Whoopee!'

Or if you have rolled 'surprised' with 'How do I sound when I feel …?', you might raise the pitch of your voice, and possibly speak more rapidly.

In a spin

This is an alternative or extension activity to 'Dicing with your emotions' for having fun at the same time as learning about the relationship between emotions and facial expressions.

Materials needed

- An empty plastic drinks bottle to act as a pointer.

- White blank cards. ('Taskmaster' blanks are excellent.)

- Coloured card, cut to business card size (using coloured card makes the game look more interesting, and differentiates between the pack of loose cards and the ones stuck on the table).

- Blu-Tack.

- Pen.

- Good solid flat table.

Making the game

You need to write the emotion words on the 'Taskmaster' (or plain white) cards. These will vary according to the ability of your clients, but could include 'happy', 'sad', 'excited', 'disgusted', 'surprised', 'tired', 'depressed', 'proud', 'in pain', 'annoyed', 'giggly', 'shocked', 'interested' and 'disapproving'.

You need to write these questions on the coloured cards:

What makes me feel …?

What does my face do when I feel …?

What might I say when I feel …?

What does my body do when I feel …?

How do I sound when I feel …?

What helps me when I feel …?

What might other people do differently from me when they feel …?

Are there times when I should not look …?

Procedure

Stick the coloured cards in a circle round the table, using the Blu-Tack, and place the empty bottle in the centre.

Take turns to pick up a loose coloured card from the stack, and then spin the bottle so that the top points towards a question. You will arrive at a question such as 'What does my face do when I feel …?', and you will have a card which says something such as 'Giggly'. The client whose turn it is should have a try at making the correct face, and if the group is amenable, others can then join in. You may have some clients in the group who need to check their facial expression in a mirror before facing the group.

Other activities to help with body language

Please see also:

1 For general work on looking, try the 'Customised Guess Who' and 'Face-out descriptions', both in Chapter 3 'Awareness of others'.

2 For getting the right 'register' or social code – when to slouch, when to sit up straight, what to wear, try the 'Formal and casual' board in Chapter 15 'Wallcharts and decorations'.

Speechmark

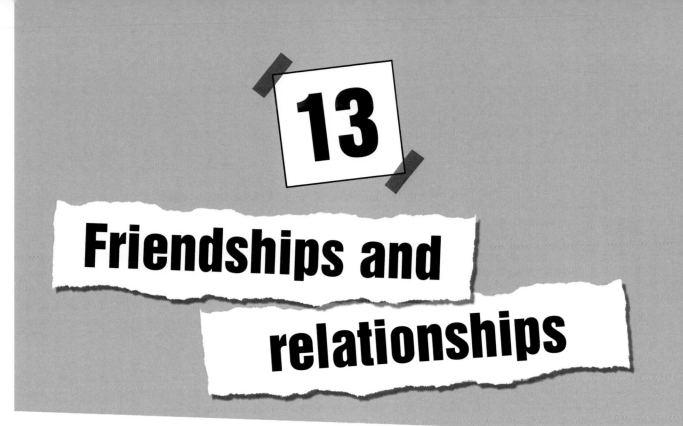

13

Friendships and relationships

If you ever learn to ski, the chances are that your instructor will tell you to tilt your weight forwards as you go downhill, rather than lean backwards, which will result in you falling back and landing on your bottom. However, every bone and sinew in your body shouts out for you to lean back because you feel that this will slow you down! Similarly, for people with friendship-making difficulties the instinct to avoid social contact is very strong, with a feeling that they will somehow be able to conjure up a girlfriend or boyfriend for life without going through the preparatory process of learning about social skills and friendship first.

Many children who have a diagnosis on the autism spectrum have difficulty in making friends, and older students and adults may also have problems in forming and maintaining relationships of various kinds, including family relationships.

The problems seem to lie in several main areas: understanding the nature and purpose of friendship; identifying potential friends; working out how to start a friendship; knowing how to maintain it; and, sometimes, how to finish it. There may also be difficulties in understanding the connections and differences between friendship and dating, and when and how to progress from one to the other.

For a deep study of the autism spectrum I thoroughly recommend Tony Attwood's books, and also those by Simon Baron-Cohen, Eric Schopler, Maxine Aston and others – please see the Bibliography at the end of this book. The ideas offered in this chapter come from my own work, and are general themes which are intended to help not only those on the spectrum, but also other clients who, for various reasons, simply have not gained much experience in forming friendships.

The outcomes of the activities are greatly improved when they are accompanied by discussion.

Talk about friendship!

It is sometimes difficult to convey the nature of friendship to people who struggle to make friends.

This activity is really a discussion forum for the meaning of friendship. The action of looking and joining up the quotes encourages reflection on the words, so is a good starting point.

You need two or three people to form a small group with you. Those who find it most useful will tend to be older teenagers and adults.

Materials needed

- Quotations about friendship, such as these:

    To have a friend be a friend.

    Make new friends but keep the old, for one is silver and the other gold.

    A friend in need is a friend indeed.

    My best friend is the one who brings out the best in me.

    A fair-weather friend.

    I get by with a little help from my friends.

    Strangers are just friends waiting to happen.

- Paper.

- Computer.

- Printer.

- Scissors.

Making the friendship cards

Print out the quotes in a fairly large font on to thick paper.

Cut the printed quotes in half.

Procedure

Each member of the group takes half a quote and looks for the other half, reads it aloud, and then discusses the meaning with the others in the group.

Extension activity

The group might like to download and print off the lyrics of songs about friendship or love. A couple of old examples you might use to demonstrate might be Carol King's 'You've Got a Friend', or Simon and Garfunkel's 'Bridge Over Troubled Water', but there are plenty of current songs that deal with the topic too.

Once you have enough examples you can use them as discussion points.

Friendship consequences

This is like the 'Consequences' game played at parties. It helps to develop awareness of others, and can be very funny when mismatches occur.

Materials needed

- Paper – which should be long and thin (A4 cut lengthways would be great as the clients will be making a long list).
- Pens.
- Paperclips.

Procedure

At the *top of the paper*, and in small writing, each participant writes about a friend (real or imaginary) to entertain and feed for a day, and regale with a gift. They should give the name and the age of the person, and indicate their preferences and dislikes for food, activities and interests. For example: 'Tyrone, aged 28, likes roast meals, hates fish, loves watching and playing football, is interested in motorbikes and is allergic to pet hair'.

This information is concealed very carefully by folding the paper over forwards twice and fixing with a paperclip. The paper is then passed on to the next player, who needs to be reminded not to unfold it. It's important to show the clients which side to write their contributions, otherwise the full text will not be in sequence at the end because some text will be on the wrong side!

The next player, not knowing the details about the 'friend' for whom they are catering, must write down a suggested activity for the morning, fold the paper over again, and pass it to the next. This player adds their idea for lunch, and folds and passes as before.

Add an afternoon activity, an idea for supper and a gift, folding and passing on after each new addition.

Now open up the paper and read the order of events for the day. You may end up with an oddly incompatible series of suggestions, for example, for Tyrone the morning activity might be to join the over-60s coffee morning, then eat baby food, then attend a ballet class, then have a prawn salad, and be given a hamster.

Discuss his reactions to all of the unfortunate suggestions, and then devise the perfect alternatives together.

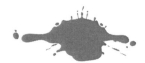

Binocular game

This is a group activity that promotes awareness of other people, and of social context. It also encourages appropriateness of conversational topic choice.

Materials needed

- Large piece of firm cardboard for the base of your game.
- Two cardboard tubes – halved kitchen paper roll centres will be fine.
- Ribbon.
- Plenty of magazine pictures of people with different backgrounds.
- Paste.
- Scissors.
- Black paint.

Making your game

You may need to cut out the pictures yourself, or your clients can, depending on their dexterity.

Stick the pictures all over the cardboard base. You don't need to leave any gaps, and it doesn't matter if they overlap a little. Try to create the effect of a crowd of people, or a party.

Link the cardboard tubes with the ribbon, but leave about 6cm between the two tubes. The idea is not to look through both 'lenses' at the same time, but to single out two separate people on the board.

For a superior effect, paint the tubes black. You may feel the need to cut them down a bit – to around 10cm.

Procedure

Each client takes a turn to place one 'lens' over the image of one person on the base board, and the other over another image.

Ask the client a series of questions such as:

What does each person look like?

Do their clothes suggest any particular interests?

How might they introduce themselves to each other?

What might they go on to talk about?

Will they become friends?

Everyone discusses the answers, with the 'observer' taking the lead and having the final say. Play then passes to the next person.

Plenty more fish in the sea

This is a humorous game about relationships, for teens and upwards. It is also a good way to introduce the concept of 'Plenty more fish in the sea' for those who keep being disappointed by their dates.

Materials needed

- Large piece of firm cardboard (better still is mountboard, which you can sometimes get from picture framers' shops if it is slightly damaged, which won't matter to you as you are going to cover it). This is for the base of your game, painted blue, and perhaps with some fish, seaweed and rocks drawn or painted on to it to add to the seaside effect.

- Small magnets with holes (obtainable from craft shops) and 30cm lengths of string – tied through the magnet holes.

- Paperclips, cards (business card blanks are ideal) and magazine pictures of different types of people. Stick a picture of one person on to each card and clip it with a paperclip (you might need to sandwich the paperclip between the picture and a plain piece of paper). You need pictures of males and females of types such as:

– Intense-looking scientists	– Students	– Walkers or hikers
– Artists	– Models	– Clergy
– Business people	– Sportspeople	Librarians
– Farmers	– Goths	– Pet lovers
– Nautical folk	– Pop singers	– DIY enthusiasts
– Doctors and nurses	– Musicians	– Cyclists.

You can add as many more types as you can think of or get pictures to represent. You need a selection of about 20–30 people.

You could also use the Speechmark ColorCards 'Occupations' set, but make sure that the magnets are capable of supporting these comparatively heavy cards, and put in an equal number of pictures of males and females.

Procedure

Place all the cards upside down on the 'sea'. Ask your clients to describe their ideal partner for a date. They hold a 'fishing line' and catch a person. The chances are that the person they catch will not match their ideal; however, they have to 'map out' a conversation with that person before thinking of a way to move on to someone else.

They need to give an idea of how they would greet that person, which topics they might talk about, questions they might ask, comments or compliments they might give, and ways of either drawing the conversation to a close, or suggesting how they might meet again.

 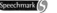

Wedding cake

This is a group activity that is particularly liked by teenage girls, but can equally well be used by boys, and can be used for both gay and straight relationships. It promotes good dating skills by encouraging appropriateness of conversational topic choice. It sets out to be light-hearted and does not intend to recommend marriage as a necessary or desirable goal! The game is related to the 'Binocular game', reinforcing some of the same skills, but presenting them in a new way.

Materials needed

- Large piece of firm cardboard, hardboard or mountboard for the base of your game. This needs to be really good and flat as you are going to use it as a sort of 'shove ha'penny' board. It also needs to be a bit bigger than your table, or if that's not possible, you will need to move it so that one side of the board can hang slightly over the table edge, and then turn it mid-game so that the other side can hang over.

- Plenty of magazine pictures of men and women as dating candidates. (Pictures of just the head and torso are fine, or you can use whole bodies if you can find good photos.) You can use photos of celebrities, and of unknown people. Have some really unlikely looking candidates, and make sure to include a few men and a few women on both sides, so that there is no heterosexual bias.

- Pictures of wedding cakes (wedding magazines often contain lots of these). Or you can draw your own cakes of different types.

- Pictures of cups of tea or coffee (again, draw your own if you can).

- Labels saying 'Never mind, try again'.

- Paste.

- Some 2p coins.

- Question document – please see below.

Making your game

You may need to cut out the pictures yourself, or your clients can, depending on their dexterity. If you are having home-drawn cakes and cups of tea, let everyone design one. The same with the 'Never mind, try again' sticky labels – everyone can write one.

Stick the pictures of the men, also a few women, along one side of the board, at the very edge, and the ladies and a few men similarly along the opposite side. Have the tops of the heads towards the outer edge. You don't need to leave any gaps along the edges, and it doesn't matter if they overlap a little. You now have a large piece of board, with lines of women and men on opposite sides, and a gap between them.

Stick the wedding cake pictures in a line right along the middle, dividing the lines of people, so there are now three parallel lines of pictures. In the intervening gaps on either side of the cakes, stick a few pictures of cups of tea, and some 'Never mind, try again' labels.

Procedure

Taking turns as 'matchmaker', choose either a man or a woman, and place a coin on that person, with a portion of the coin hanging over the edge of the board. With the flat of your hand, give the coin a sharp shove, so that it travels across the board to a person on the other side.

Now your clients need to answer a series of questions:

What does each person say to the other, to start the conversation?

What do they go on to talk about?

What do they agree about, and where do they disagree?

Do you think they will go on a date? If yes, where might they go for this date?

Now the group must discuss whether, given the facts, the couple are likely to make good partners. If they think the matchmaker has made out a good case for a lifelong commitment between their candidates, then the matchmaker can choose and describe one of the cake pictures.

If the group cannot decide whether the couple are sufficiently matched then the group will opt for the 'Cup of tea' option, and can go on to discuss what else the potential couple might need to talk about.

If it's a definite 'no' for that couple, then the 'Never mind, try again' labels are pointed at. (But the matchmaker can't have another go until it is their next turn.)

Now it's the turn of another potential matchmaker.

If many 'cakes' have been awarded, and mouths are watering, you might need to provide a real cake, or at least a biscuit, at the end of the session!

Snakes and ladders of dating

The old Victorian version of Snakes and Ladders was a sort of morality judgement. The person who won was deemed to be the most virtuous, while the loser was a low sinner! The numbers attached to the seven snakes and seven ladders related to a list of vices and virtues printed in the lid of the box.

Modern versions have more snakes and ladders on the board, usually 13 of each.

This game uses a modification of the old system as a light-hearted model for a dating game that promotes discussion.

It is great fun to play in a group, and works well with teenagers. It is very important that the texts, which are read aloud, are taken in a light-hearted manner; you don't want anyone to feel that they would really behave like that on a date. It is best to explain, before you start, that these are just pretend situations. Group members could even take assumed names for the length of the game.

Materials needed

- A Snakes and Ladders game with a dice and several counters.

- A list of successful behaviours (to go with the ladders), and a list of unsuccessful ones (to go with the snakes).

Procedure

Take turns to roll the dice and move your counter. When someone lands on the bottom of a ladder they move their counter upwards as indicated. They also read aloud the accompanying text about 'good behaviour' on a date. Similarly when someone lands at the top of a snake they have to move down to the tail, and read out the 'bad behaviour' text which goes with that.

Here are some suggestions for the behaviours, with the original numbers that link to them on most boards. It's a good idea to check that the numbers correspond with your board before trying the game; you may need to make some alterations.

Snakes

24 Vanity: you spend far too long staring at yourself in the mirror and choosing clothes.

27 Envy: while out on a date you keep talking about how another girl or boy has all the things you want, put yourself in a bad mood, and spoil the evening.

36 Anger: you can't agree on things and keep arguing.

50 Laziness: you never make an effort to look nice or try hard to make the date go well.

54 Possessiveness: you can't let them out of your sight. You don't like it if they talk to anyone else.

60 Gluttony: you eat too quickly on your date to a restaurant, and then spoil the date by being sick.

69 Lust: you go too far too fast, and it puts your partner off.

83 Drunkenness: you drink too much on a date, and that leads to you behaving badly.

88 Meanness: you never offer to pay your way on a date, so your partner can't afford to take you out so often.

90 Dishonesty: you told your date that it doesn't matter if you are late back. This gets you both into trouble.

92 Rudeness: you forget to compliment your partner and forget to say thank-you for a good evening.

95 Vulgarity: you keep burping, or worse, on the date.

99 Lateness: you keep being late for dates and meetings.

Ladders

3 Modesty: you are not out to impress just by the way you look. On a date that involves a country walk you wear the right clothes, and your walking shoes.

12 Humour: you laugh at your partner's jokes, and make some good ones of your own.

15 Chilled-ness: you don't get flustered if your partner has a different opinion. You can agree to differ.

18 Organisation: you try to make sure the day will go well; you've arranged to visit some nice places.

21 Liberality: your partner's needs are more important to you than your own. You are happy to see the film your partner wants to see, even though it's not your choice.

47 Moderation: you eat just the right amount, feeling healthy for a pleasant walk after lunch.

49 Reserve: you prefer to wait until the third date before attempting a proper kiss.

53 Temperance: you remember not to mix 'grape and grain', and are happy to have soft drinks too. You are in control this way.

57 Generosity: you offer to pay for your partner sometimes. You remember their birthday.

59 Honesty: you would never two-time your partner.

64 Politeness: you paid your partner a compliment. You said how much you enjoyed the film or outing.

72 Self-control: you needed to burp, but managed not to. You were the perfect lady or gentleman.

82 Reliability: you are always there when you say you will be.

Other activities to help with friendship building

Please see also:

1 '"How I help people" poster' in Chapter 2 'Self-awareness and self-esteem'.

2 'Friendship bands', 'Gift list' and 'Tourist information game', activities which are all in Chapter 3 'Awareness of others'.

3 'Friendship vine' in Chapter 15 'Wallcharts and decorations'.

Speechmark

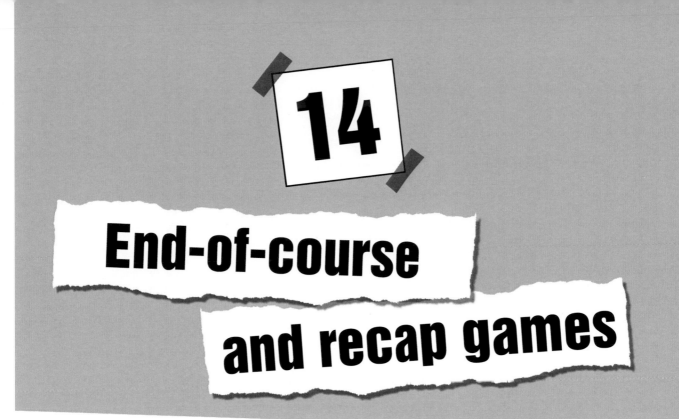

End-of-course and recap games

When you have finished a set of sessions, it rounds things off nicely if the very last session can be both light-hearted and at the same time a way of recapping on the therapy that the clients have been doing.

The best forms of recap will refer to activities previously carried out in the course of the therapy as a way of reminding clients, so a repetition of a therapy game that was enjoyed will be well received.

Aim to review the clients' achievements with them at the end of a course, so that you are able to show them where they have made improvements, and give praise. A thorough formal reassessment would not normally take place at these recap sessions, however.

Here are some suggestions for adaptable games that you can engineer to recap on anything you have tackled.

Customised Jenga

A good fun activity for a group at the end of a course of therapy. It is essential to have a solid table with a flat surface for this game, otherwise you will spend the whole session rebuilding the tower! For the same reason, only do this activity with clients who have a steady hand.

Materials needed

- A game of Jenga, or similar. If you are very enterprising or impecunious you could cut the little blocks yourself, but you would have to be fussy about sanding them thoroughly so that they will slide out of the tower easily.

- A pen with a very fine tip.

How to make your game

There are two plain sides on each Jenga block, and all you do is write 'forfeits' on them. This is easy to do; the greater task is thinking of enough forfeits.

Published games such as The Ungame, Let's Talk or All About Me might give you inspiration for some ideas for your blocks, or you can make the ideas up yourself. It is helpful to have forfeits of different types, for example, category areas such as 'My favourite food' or 'Name three farm animals', as well as more philosophical ones such as 'If I won a million pounds I would …' or 'If I had a time-travel machine I would go …' Also give some social skill types such as 'Greet everyone in the group in a different way' or 'What would you do if your friend was in a bad mood?' and some 'silly' ones such as 'Walk round the table like an old lady' or 'Make a noise like a chicken'.

Procedure

Play as for ordinary Jenga, but after you have pulled out a brick you have to carry out the forfeit. There is a forfeit on each side, making a choice. I have had no trouble with the same forfeit coming up more than once in a session, because there are no right answers to the questions, so you can have several people's thoughts on the same subject.

The one who knocks the tower down has the job of rebuilding it!

Variations

If you want to target a particular skill – phonology, let's say, or body language – you will need to have another set of bricks from which you take a few for each 'add-on' skill. Write on instructions pertaining to that skill, and then mix them in with your standard set, removing the same number of your standard ones so that you don't have a hugely tall tower that could form a safety hazard! For ease of sorting, colour the ends of the 'specialist skills' bricks with felt tips, for example, phonology red, body language blue and ambiguity orange.

End-of-course board game

Here is another way to remind clients of the contents of the course they have completed. It is a multi-use board game and will give you many opportunities for activities if you make it sturdily. It is best for a group of young clients, but depending on the instructions you use, and the design of the board, you can apply it to other age groups too.

Materials needed

- A3 size card, paper, or a large piece of felt or other fabric.
- Small sticky labels.
- Sticky stars or coloured dots.
- Small cards (business card blanks or 'Taskmaster' cards).
- Pen and felt tips.
- Stapler or superglue, if you are using a piece of felt as your background.
- Decoration for the board if it is paper or card, for example, football, car, celebrity or fashion pictures, from magazines, or you and your clients could draw your own design.
- Glue.
- A dice and playing pieces (you could use coins for the pieces if you have nothing else available).

Making your game

You or your clients need to decorate the background for the board game – it could be a drawing of a jungle, a seaside image, a house, and so on, or a collection of images from magazines to be stuck on. We used a large piece of felt (part of the green baize from a discarded billiard table) to make a Christmas tree shape for the end of the Christmas term.

Stick on your sticky labels, say 25–30 of them, and number them logically and off-centre so that there is room beside the number for a sticker. Decide on your route around the board, making it end at a special point (the route around our felt tree ended at the top). If you are using fabric you will need to use staples or superglue to keep the labels on. Stick a star or a dot towards the side of every second or third number – these will be the points at which a card is taken and the instructions followed. Try to have about 10 –15 of these stopping points.

Write on the cards the instructions that are appropriate to the work you have been doing – a listening task, some phonology challenges, an idiom to define. You will need plenty of instruction cards, more than the number of stopping points.

Procedure

This is a simple 'roll the dice and move that number of spaces' type of game. Whenever a stopping point is reached an instruction card is turned over and the task followed.

End-of-course recap cards

These are good for reminders of the course content, without being as formal as homework. They also add to parents' information of what their child has been learning about.

Materials needed

- A4 size blank card (coloured if you like).
- A5 envelopes.
- Pen and felt tips.
- Access to a photocopier.

Making your cards

For one group of clients:

Choose, for the front of your clients' cards, a simple and appropriate outline that is relevant to the school term, or to the client's interests. Draw, for example, a sun with rays, or a Christmas tree, an egg shape, a heraldic shield, the outline of a Dalek, or something else. (There are lots of outline images available for free downloading from the internet.)

As the therapist you will decide what to add to the shape; you would write inside and around it the topics covered during that phase of work. For example, you could write 'Body language' inside the Christmas tree, and add the words 'Eye contact', 'Smiling', 'Waving', 'High fives' and 'Handshake' as baubles on the branches.

Add any decorations you want to include, and then photocopy for each member of the group. Keep a copy for yourself, as you might have a similar group another time!

Fold the pieces of card to make them A5 sized, to fit the envelopes.

Your clients could add colours before they take their cards home.

Spin the bottle

This type of activity must be the best value ever! Its possibilities are only limited by your imagination, and it costs next to nothing.

Materials needed

- One empty plastic drink bottle.
- Sheets of sticky labels.
- A table with a forgiving surface.
- Pens.

Completing the bottle

Write the labels appropriately for what you have been working on, for example:

For a recap of 'Vocabulary' you could revisit category work. In which case you would need to write the different categories on the labels, and stick them in a large circle on the table, or for opposites you might write one of the halves of opposite pairs.

For a recap of 'Lateral thinking' you might write names of items on the labels, for clients to think of alternative uses for them.

For 'Body language' you might write labels with emotions on them, for the clients to make the appropriate face that goes with the emotion.

Procedure

Your clients sit around the table and take turns to spin the bottle, naming things in the nearest category pointed to by the bottle when it stops.

Variations

1 You could write or illustrate words for sign language practice.

2 You could write letters of the alphabet on the labels, for participants to think of a word beginning with that sound.

3 I have also used this game for 're-bonding' a group after a longish break. The labels I wrote were:

Since last time, I've been to …

Since last time, I've met …

'Since last time, I've learnt …

Since last time, I've made …

Since last time, something that was on the news …

Since last time, something that changed for me was …

Other ideas for end-of-course and recap games

Please see also:

1 'Butterfly game' in Chapter 11 'Motivating your clients', tweaking it slightly to focus on the area of work you are trying to recap.

2 The seasonal (Christmas) variation on '"Also for ..."' in Chapter 7 'Lateral thinking' if the recap session is at the end of the Christmas term.

3 'Tourist information game' in Chapter 3 'Awareness of others' if your recap session is at the end of the summer term.

4 'Communication tree' in Chapter 15 'Wallcharts and decorations' for an end of Social Skills course.

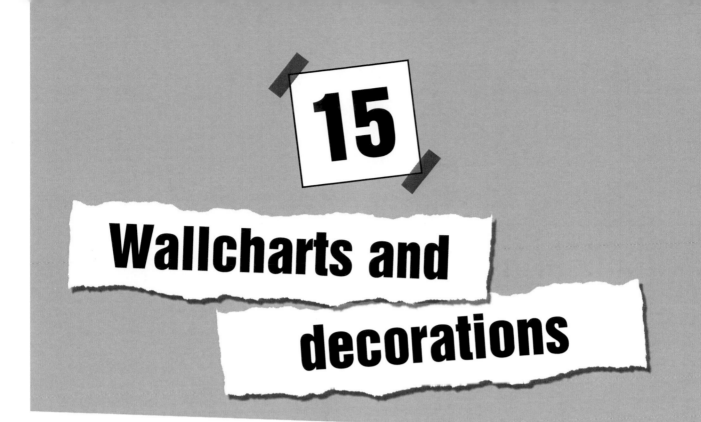

15

Wallcharts and decorations

Do you sometimes feel you would like to improve the look of your therapy room? I have worked in many odd SLT spaces over the years; one was strongly reminiscent of a Nissen hut, another had been a cricket pavilion, another, a cellar. In one hospital the SLT room was almost entirely beige – the walls, notice board, curtains, seat covers and filing cabinet, with one item camouflaging the next!

Such a neutral scheme is the perfect solution for clients who are distractible, or for those who cannot abide particular colours. Some on the autism spectrum, for example, may not be able to tolerate bright colours or lots of posters. On the other hand, some clients (and you) may find a lack of colour a boring prospect, even depressing, and, for those who have some degree of visual impairment, a room that is all one colour can be difficult to navigate around.

A good compromise seems to be to have a fairly soothing neutral background, but one which is enhanced by posters and other decorations. Distractible clients are often comfortable with these if they have been involved in some way with the making process.

Here are some ideas for adding to your walls something that is related to your therapy, or to the seasons. They are easy for you and your clients to make, although some are better if partly prepared beforehand.

'Formal and casual' board

This is a wall-mounted display for a group to make. It helps clients learn about the various 'social codes' needed for different situations. It is good fun to create, and forms the basis for many discussions.

Materials needed

- As many newspaper or magazine pictures as you can find, depicting people in different social contexts, for example, at barbecues, weddings, legal trials and dances. (I've found that, as a general rule, local papers are a good source of photos of 'casual' events, while the nationals, especially broadsheets, tend to yield more 'formal' images.)

- Large board (either a piece of hardboard about 1m by 1.5m, or a large pinboard with a frame, obtainable from DIY shops or stationers).

- Glue or pins, felt tips, scissors.

- Post-it notes: some ordinary ones, and some speech bubble ones.

- Acrylic varnish.

Making the board

Write the word 'Formal' on a sticker at the top of the board and similarly 'Casual' at the bottom, and try to leave these stickers visible as you proceed.

Completing the board

The clients cut out the pictures and arrange them on the board, deciding between them how far up towards the formal or down towards the casual they should be placed. It's best not to stick them until all of the cards have been arranged, to allow for changes of mind! You should end up with a bottom row of casual images such as a group of people in a pub, on a beach or at a barbecue or picnic. Then, working upwards, there will be several rows of progressively more formal images, including scenes such as shopping, school, college or work, cafés, doctors' waiting rooms and appointments, until you reach the pictures showing formal settings, for example, courtroom scenes, passing-out parades, funerals and state banquets (they don't have to be situations the clients have actually experienced; in fact the more extreme the better.)

If you have time, it would make the whole thing much sturdier if you could varnish it with a layer of acrylic varnish. The edges will stay down much better and it will withstand Post-it notes being applied to it and pulled off again.

Now to relate the levels of formality to the clients' lives. Each client writes, on a Post-it note, a short sentence about an occasion they have been to, and put it in the right place according to its formality level. Situations might include: going to the snooker hall; work experience at the garden centre; phoning home; phoning Mum's office; texting a friend;

visiting an older relative; going to a wedding; or a Duke of Edinburgh's award ceremony.

Discussion points would be whether, for example, phoning Mum's office is more or less formal than asking for something in a shop.

Extras and variations

Add little speech bubble Post-it notes to the pictures with greetings set at the appropriate level, that is, ranging from 'Hi' to 'Morning' to 'Good morning'. If you write these on Post-it notes you can vary the type of bubble to include farewells and conversational topics.

Discuss, and possibly write on the poster, appropriate forms of non-verbal greetings, for example, 'High fives', handshakes, salutes, even curtsies!

You could also discuss appropriate clothing for each scenario, types of food that might be served, or which music could be played.

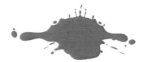

Communication tree

This has been a really useful collage item to have on the wall of the clinic. It helps with motivation and understanding the interactive process. It is useful at the early stages of a social language group, where the clients are beginning to be aware of the skills they could improve in order to become better communicators, and is also a handy end-of-course recap.

You are aiming to create an outline image of a tree, with roots and branches, to which the clients can attach leaf-shaped labels describing the ways in which communication benefits us, and earth clod-shaped labels stating prerequisites for achieving good communication. In other words, the leaves of the tree represent the outcomes of being a good communicator, while the roots explain which areas we need to work on in order to become good at communicating.

You will need to have constructed the base before your clients complete it. It is worth making the basic framework sturdily, because you can then use it again and again. Alternatively, you could make it out of paper as a quick illustrative exercise.

It may take the group more than one session to complete the tree.

Materials needed

- A piece of board – A2 size is about right. Fibreboard is ideal as you can stick pins into it. It's best to use it portrait way round.

- Pale blue fabric to cover the whole board. Old polycotton sheeting is fine for this.

- Beige fabric to cover the lower third of the board – representing the area under the ground where roots form.

- Thin strip of greenish fabric to form a 'grass level'.

- Rough-textured brown fabric. We used hessian with success as it is textured enough to resemble tree bark and roots, yet lightweight enough to stay stuck to the backing.

- Glue (PVA is good as it doesn't show through the fabric, and will wash off clients' clothes).

- Leaf-green paper (several shades of green would be great).

- Earthy-brown paper.

- Pens, scissors and pins.

Preparing the board

Stick the blue fabric on the board to cover it completely and add the beige across the bottom third, forming the earth.

Draw your tree on the textured brown fabric and cut it out. It's a good idea to make it a many-branched variety so that you will have lots of room for leaf and clod labels. Don't worry if you can't cut out the root part at the same time, as you can cover the join with 'grass' anyway. Stick your tree on, and stick the grass across where the roots meet the trunk, and the earth meets the sky. Write the word 'COMMUNICATION' on or alongside the trunk. Now you have the basic form to which your clients can attach labels.

Completing the board

It is important that you discuss with your clients the reasons for making the board, and I have found that it is best to begin with the subject of the benefits of being able to communicate. The clients will tell you why it is important, but you should end up with a list including the following: chatting to people; making friends; using the phone; making appointments; asking for things in shops; telling people what you need; making jokes; having discussions; being part of a group; interview skills; getting a girl- or boyfriend and keeping in touch with old acquaintances.

Write down all the suggestions as they are given, and then give everyone in the group some green paper and scissors to cut out leaves to stick on the tree. The tendency is for people to cut leaves that are too small to write on, so suggest that they write first, then cut them out and pin them on the tree.

Now you need to tackle the roots of the tree in a similar way, first discussing the prerequisites for good communication and making a list, this time including skills such as listening, body language, speech clarity, eye contact, using the person's name, greetings and farewells, turn taking, being optimistic, staying on or shifting the subject, having a few topics ready, prioritising and organising.

It is likely that several of these areas will be unfamiliar to your clients, especially the areas that are not a problem to them, so you will need to give an outline description; however, you are not actually teaching these skills at this stage.

Again, make the suggestions into labels and pin them to the tree, this time using clod shapes, at the roots.

Discussion

Ask everyone how they feel about the tree, and which bits apply to them. Discuss how real trees use their roots to draw nourishment from the earth, and can therefore put out shoots. Try to make the point really clearly that if they work at the prerequisite skills they will be able to reap the benefits.

Totem pole

A fun activity, which is useful for a teenage social language group. The result is quite a large cylindrical object, about 1.5m tall, so bear this in mind before you start, if your therapy room is small.

Native American people's totem poles depict animals that reflect or encourage aspects of their culture and personalities. We made a cardboard one that was designed to encourage various conversation skills. Perhaps not quite so aesthetically pleasing as the original carved wood variety, but this calls on a cooperative approach and results in a big object with impact!

Materials needed

- You need a cardboard tube with as big a diameter as possible. We obtained one that had been the centre of a carpet roll, and cut off a 1.5m length. The actual cutting is quite a job, and needs a bit of muscle and a saw (ie you can't do this with a pair of scissors).
- Large sheets of strong paper in shades of brown.
- Felt tips, scissors and glue.
- String and parcel tape.
- Sticky labels.
- Drill (optional).

Making the totem pole

First you need to talk through the aspects of conversation that you are hoping to target. The group should already be aware of the meaning of terminology such as 'eye contact', 'listening skills', 'topic maintenance (or focus)', 'body language' and 'turn taking'.

Decide on animals that could be associated with each conversation skill. We chose an owl for eye contact, a bat for listening, a heron for topic maintenance or focus and a peacock for body language (admittedly from the wrong continent, but an excellent example of animal body language, and one that they all knew). For turn taking we added a paper 'talking stick'* half way down, but you could demonstrate poor turn taking, by adding a pig – not noted for polite turn taking at the trough!

Once the length of the pole has been cut, you need to fix tying points so that you will be able to attach your finished pole to a wall. We stuck lengths of string round the pole, but you could drill pairs of holes with string through instead. In either case, don't scrimp on the lengths of string you allow to hang out, and make sure you have aligned them to correspond with attachment points in your room.

* The 'talking stick' is described on page 54 in Chapter 5 'Conversation skills'.

Now you need to draw the animals on to the paper – each client can be in charge of a particular animal. The trick is to keep the drawings tall, so that they will just overlap when stuck to the pole, and be the right size to cover the perimeter of the pole.

The finished effect of the pole will be enhanced if, when you cut out the animals, you allow ears, wings and beaks to protrude, by careful cutting round the shapes. Glue them to the pole, leaving your strings out.

Attach the pole to the wall using the strings.

Stick labels that name the animal and describe the conversation skill connection either on each animal, or on the wall beside your pole.

Make sure you create opportunities to discuss and possibly role play examples of good conversational techniques.

Speechmark

Friendship vine

This is another useful collage item to have on the wall of the clinic. It promotes understanding of the process of forming friendships.

You are aiming to create an outline image of a grapevine, with roots, branches and leaves, to which the clients can attach labels in the shape of bunches of grapes, describing the ways in which friendships benefit us, and other labels in the shape of clods of earth, stating prerequisites for achieving friendships.

You will need to have constructed the base before your clients complete it. It is worth making the basic framework sturdily if you think you would use it again. I have described how to make a fabric version of the vine, as it lasts a long time and doesn't reflect light. Alternatively, you could make it out of paper as a quick illustrative exercise, in which case you would substitute paints for the fabric areas.

It may take the group more than one session to complete the vine.

Materials needed

- A piece of board – A2 size is about right. Fibreboard is ideal as you can stick pins into it. It's best to use it landscape way round.

- Pale blue fabric to cover the whole board. Old polycotton sheeting is fine for this.

- Beige fabric to cover the lower third of the board – representing the area under the ground where roots form.

- Thin strip of greenish fabric to form a 'grass level'.

- Brown fabric – for the vine's trunk, branches and roots.

- Glue (PVA is good as it doesn't show through the fabric).

- Leaf-green fabric (several shades of green would be great).

- Purple paper for the grape bunch labels (not too dark, as you will be writing on them).

- Earthy-brown paper for the clod of earth labels.

- Pens, scissors and pins.

Preparing the board

Stick the blue fabric on the board to cover it completely and add the beige across the bottom third, forming the earth.

Draw your vine on the brown fabric and cut it out. It's a good idea to make it a long-branched variety so that you will have lots of room for the bunches of grapes, also leaving room for the clods of earth. Stick your vine on, and stick the grass across where the roots meet the trunk, and the earth meets the sky. Write the word 'FRIENDSHIP' along the trunk. Now you have the basic form to which your clients can attach labels.

Speechmark

Completing the board

It is important that you discuss with your clients the reasons for making the board, and begin with the subject of the benefits of being able to make friends (follow up with the 'How to make friends' part later).

The clients should tell you why friendship is important, but you will probably end up with a list including the following: company, for example, when going out; someone to talk to; someone to share things and ideas with; someone to 'take your side'; someone to send you a postcard; someone to remember your birthday; someone to give you support when you are feeling depressed and someone to try out jokes on.

Write down all the suggestions as they are given, and then give everyone in the group some purple paper and scissors to cut out bunches of grapes to stick on the tree. The tendency is for people to cut shapes that are too small to write on, so suggest to them that they write first, then cut them out and pin them on the vine.

Now you need to tackle the roots of the vine in a similar way, first discussing the foundations and responsibilities for friendship forming. Make a list, this time including such ideas as being cheerful, providing support, being loyal, being trustworthy, sharing and keeping secrets. Other 'roots' will mention skills such as going to places where potential friends might be, joining in, talking, recognising a true friend.

It is likely that several of these areas will be unfamiliar to your clients, especially the areas that are not a problem to them, so you will need to give an outline description; however, you are not actually teaching these skills at this stage.

Again make the suggestions into labels and pin them to the vine, this time using clod shapes, at the roots.

Discussion

Ask everyone how they feel about the vine, and which bits apply to them. Discuss how real vines use their roots to draw nourishment from the earth, and can therefore produce grapes.

Try to make the point really clearly that if the clients work at the prerequisite skills they will be able to reap the benefits.

Arty party

This activity works well for clients who like humour, and especially for anyone interested in art. However, they must not mind having famous artwork 'enhanced' by a few additions! It was designed to help people who need to develop their skills at conversational comments, or jokey one-liners. It also encourages clients to look carefully at faces, for their emotional expressions, and at images, for details.

It makes an interesting wall decoration that can be added to over several weeks. You can use it with a group, where the benefit is that ideas can be sparked off each other, often causing much mirth, or you can try it in the one-to-one setting where a client will have more time to think of a witticism in peace.

Materials needed

- A sheet of paper (flipchart paper is fine), or use a notice board.

- Images of artworks that depict two or more people. You can sometimes find these in colour supplements that feature a particular artist or artistic movement. Other good sources are museums and art galleries where they sell artists' postcards. Alternatively you could just use colour photos from colour supplements.

- Post-it notes in the shape of speech bubbles (from stationers).

- Pens.

- Glue or Blu-Tack.

Preparing the background

Try to find images in which the people have different facial expressions, for example, one serious, the other surprised or pleading. Or you might find an image with one person laughing while the other looks angry, sad or bored. Also look for examples where there is an odd or amusing detail. It's best to avoid anything religious.

Select an image with a person who seems to you to be making a comment, and another who you can imagine giving an amusing (but not rude) riposte, and write these comments on two Post-it notes. Stick the picture on to the backing paper and apply the speech bubbles.

Now you have an example that will, if you have managed to make a funny comment, encourage your clients. For a bit of background inspiration, look at satirical shows on TV, and listen to the kinds of comments about photos of politicians made by comedians. In the therapy setting it's probably wise to avoid politicians, though!

Procedure

It is important that you discuss the images and the point of the exercise with your clients, and that you give them plenty of time to select an image that they can enhance with their ideas for speech bubbles. They might even prefer to take an image away with them and add their comments at home, then bring them to the following therapy session.

Once they are happy with an image and their response to it, they can stick it (or Blu-Tack it) to the paper. Random spacing and angle of placement often give a more effective look.

Leave this wall decoration up, with a selection of appropriate images and Post-it notes nearby, because other clients may see it and wish to add to it.

Discussion and development

Discuss the result together and aim to have a laugh at everyone's efforts.

Make the point that it is not a good idea to laugh at the expense of a friend, although politicians and imaginary characters are perhaps fair game.

Fields of interest

Here is a practical way of registering the interests and hobbies of clients in a college or school, so that they can meet others with similar ideas – potentially forming new friendships in this way. The clients' names should be put on the register if they are happy to let many people know that they have a genuine interest in an area already listed, or if they would like to start a new one. They should be prepared to accept that they might be unique in their interest. The clients will also learn the meaning of the expression 'field of interest'.

It is nice if the 'fields' can be wall mounted, but if this is not possible, they could be in a notebook or file.

Materials needed

- The largest Post-it notes you can get, or if you have a notice board or wall space you can pin or Blu-Tack ordinary paper up. Green is the ideal colour, if you can get it, as it is more field-like.

- A sheet of flipchart paper to attach the fields to, and headed with the title 'Fields of Interest' (or just 'Our Interests' if you prefer).

- I have also found a plastic pocketed wall hanging for displaying postcards useful – more expensive, but neater and easier to move (obtainable from Habitat and other such shops). For this version you just buy blank postcards to write on and put in the pockets.

Procedure

Ask clients about their interests, and start a few of the lists, heading each Post-it note with the name of the interest, fascination or hobby and adding their name underneath. Interests could be anything from basketball to cookery, or a particular type of music. If you are working with people on the autism spectrum, be prepared for some unusual interests such as disposal skip firms, train timetables or a fondness for collecting electrical plugs.

Encourage the next group of clients to spend time thinking about the 'Fields of Interest' sheets, and let them add their names underneath those already there, or start new fields.

Once you have a pair or more of people with a shared interest, you may find that they already know each other, but had not discovered the similar interest. However, they may need to be introduced for the first time.

It will be up to the clients to decide how to proceed, for example, whether they would like to have a trip together to an electrical supplier. It may be enough for them just to know that they are not alone in their unusual fascination or, on the other hand, that so far they are the one and only waste skip enthusiast.

If you have many non-reading clients you can head the lists with small symbols (Widgit symbols for preference, if those are the types the clients are already used to, or Clipart ones).

Interaction paper chains for Christmas

A simple and festive idea to recap on work done in the pre-Christmas period, and a way to link all your various clients and groups together.

You are aiming to create festive decorations on which the clients have written down ways in which communication benefits us, or prerequisites for achieving good communication. Friendship and social skills and conversation tips can all be included as well.

Materials needed

- Packs of coloured paper strips sold for Christmas decorations. These are sold already glued at one end. Avoid the metallic variety as you won't be able to write on them so easily.

- Pens.

Procedure

Each client writes one aspect of communication on a strip. Ideally the aspect they choose would be something on their personal target list for the term. They can work on as many strips as they like, to make a long chain; you need to make it look like an intended decoration rather than a timid little offering! Make sure you keep back some unwritten strips, so that you can eventually use them at the ends of each chain as attachment points.

Curl one strip round, and stick it to itself to form a paper circle, then loop another through it, and so on until you have a long chain which can be added to, by other groups or individuals. Don't hang your chain too high, because you need to be able to see the words written on the loops.

Discussion

Ask everyone how they feel about the chain, and which targets belonging to other clients might also apply to them.

Other ideas for wallcharts and clinic decorations

Please see also:

1 '"How I help people" poster' in Chapter 2 'Self-awareness and self-esteem'.

2 'Paint splotch predictions', also in Chapter 2 'Self-awareness and self-esteem'.

3 '"Same and different" chains', also in Chapter 2 'Self-awareness and self-esteem'.

4 'Standing in your shoes' in Chapter 3 'Awareness of others'.

speechmark

Bibliography and recommended further reading

Self-awareness and self-esteem

Fitzpatrick P, Clarke K & Higgins P (1994) *Self-Esteem*, The Chalkface Project.

Lear E (2002) *The Complete Nonsense and Other Verse*, Penguin.

McGough R & Brandreth G (eds) (1999) *The Big Book of Little Poems*, Andre Deutsch.

Sunderland M & Englehart P (1997) *Draw On Your Emotions*, Speechmark.

Awareness of others

Gajewski N, Hirn P & Mayo P (1998) *Social Skills Strategies*, Books A and B, Thinking Publications.

Listening skills

Leslie C & Crewdson D (2006) *Working With Listening Problems* (course).

Conversation skills

Alexander M (1995) 'Big talk, small talk: BT takes a look at British telephone culture', paper presented to MRS Conference, London.

Lowndes L (1999) *How to Talk to Anyone*, Thorsons.

Rinaldi W (n.d.) *Language Choices* (course and manual).

Townsend S (1983) *The Secret Diary of Adrian Mole Aged 13¾*, Methuen.

Speech sound production

Gorrie B & Parkinson E (1995) *Phonological Awareness Activity*, Stass Publications.

Lewis S (2004) *Talking Phonology*, Bird Art Publications.

For more ideas on staff training on understanding phonology difficulties, please see the chapter on 'Augmentative communication' in a clip file which is also useful for a host of other training ideas:

Thurman S, Stewart K & Jones J (1991) *Talking Points*, Stass Publications.

Lateral thinking

Borthwick C (1993) *Semantic Topics: Divergent Thinking Activities,* Stass Publications.

Burningham J (1978) *Would You Rather?*, Jonathan Cape.

Memory

Dohrmann V (1994) *Treating Memory Impairments*, Communication Skill Builders.

Rinaldi W (n.d.) *Social Use of Language Programme*.

Vocabulary

Buzan T & Buzan B (2009) *The Mind Map Book*, BBC Active.

Lewis S (2004) *Semantic Steps*, Bird Art Publications.

Ambiguity

Bromberger O (1997) *Turn Me Round*, Tobar Ltd.

Escher M C (2008) *The Graphic Work*, Taschen.

Hanks M (2004) *The Ultimate Book of Incredible Eye Twisters*, Metro Publishing.

Jack A (2004) *Red Herrings and White Elephants: The Origins of the Phrases We Use Every Day*, Metro Publishing.

Lakoff G & Johnson M (2003) *Metaphors We Live By*, University of Chicago Press (this edition contains a good 'Afterword').

Legler D (1991) *Don't Take it so Literally!*, ECL Publications.

Lewis S, Hunt L & Papier T (1998) *Mystifying Metaphors and Smiley Similes*, Bird Art Publications.

Rothstein J & Gooding M (1999) *The Playful Eye*, Redstone Press.

Seckel A (2002) *The Fantastic World of Optical Illusions*, Carlton Books.

Seckel A (2007) *Incredible Visual Illusions*, Arcturus Publishing.

Stuart-Hamilton I (2004) *An Asperger Dictionary of Everyday Expressions*, Jessica Kingsley.

Body language

Baron-Cohen S (2004) *Mind Reading* (CD Rom), Jessica Kingsley.

Clayton P (2003) *Body Language at Work*, Hamlyn.

McConnell N & LoGuidice C (1998) *That's Life! Social Language*, LinguiSystems.

Pease A (1997) *Body Language*, 3rd edn, Sheldon Press.

Friendships and relationships

Aston M (2003) *Aspergers in Love: Couple Relationships and Family Affairs*, Jessica Kingsley.

Edmonds G & Worton D (2005) *The Asperger Love Guide*, Paul Chapman.

Generally useful throughout this book, and recommended for further reading

Attwood T (2007) *The Complete Guide to Asperger's Syndrome*, Jessica Kingsley.

Berger S & Hawkins G (2006) *Ready Made*, Thames & Hudson.

Jackson L (2002) *Freaks, Geeks and Asperger Syndrome: A User Guide to Adolescence*, Jessica Kingsley.

Kelly A (1997) *Talkabout: A Social Communication Skills Package*, Speechmark.

Messibor G B, Shea V & Schopler E (2004) *The TEACCH Approach to Autism Spectrum Disorders*, Plenum.

Index of activities